Virtual Patient Encounters
for
Aehlert:
Paramedic Practice Today: Above and Beyond

Virtual Patient Encounters

for

Aehlert: Paramedic Practice Today: Above and Beyond

Study Guide prepared by

Jon Cooper, NREMT-P
Lieutenant
Baltimore City Fire and EMS Academy
Baltimore, Maryland

Steven Dralle, BA, LP
Product Marketing Manager
Vidacare
San Antonio, Texas

Larry Richmond, AS, NREMT-P, CCEMT-P
EMS Education Manager
Mountain Plains Health Consortium
Fort Meade, South Dakota

Software developed by

Wolfsong Informatics, LLC
Tucson, Arizona

MOSBY JEMS

ELSEVIER

MOSBY JEMS
ELSEVIER

11830 Westline Industrial Drive
St. Louis, Missouri 63146

VIRTUAL PATIENT ENCOUNTERS   ISBN: 978-0-323-04920-7
FOR AEHLERT: PARAMEDIC PRACTICE TODAY:
ABOVE AND BEYOND

Notice

Knowledge and best practice in this field are constantly changing. As new research and experience broaden our knowledge, changes in practice, treatment and drug therapy may become necessary or appropriate. Readers are advised to check the most current information provided (i) on procedures featured or (ii) by the manufacturer of each product to be administered, to verify the recommended dose or formula, the method and duration of administration, and contraindications. It is the responsibility of the practitioner, relying on their own experience and knowledge of the patient, to make diagnoses, to determine dosages and the best treatment for each individual patient, and to take all appropriate safety precautions. To the fullest extent of the law, neither the Publisher nor the Author assumes any liability for any injury and/or damage to persons or property arising out or related to any use of the material contained in this book.

ISBN: 978-0-323-04920-7

Vice President and Publisher: Andrew Allen
Executive Editor: Linda Honeycutt
Editor: Scott Weaver
Publishing Services Manager: Trish Tannian
Project Manager: Jonathan M. Taylor
Cover Designer: Amy Buxton

Printed in the United States of America

Last digit is the print number: 9 8 7 6 5 4 3 2 1

Contents

*Summative lesson—see "Orientation to *Virtual Patient Encounters*" for explanation.

Summative Lessons Listed by Case

Acknowledgments

Virtual Patient Encounters was developed with input from many emergency medical services (EMS) instructors around the United States who participated in some fashion. Some traveled across the country to share their vision of what a valuable critical-thinking product would be; others wrote cases and recommended management sequences; some provided their expertise at focus groups and user-centered design studies; and many instructors reviewed the software, study guide, and implementation manual.

We are deeply grateful to each of you for helping us make this implementation manual a reality. Your education, dedication, and experience clearly shine through in this one-of-a-kind educational product for paramedic students everywhere. Recognizing your contributions wherever you were involved— in the software, the study guide, and/or the implementation manual—does not truly express our gratitude.

I would like to offer a special thank you to three of the best instructors in EMS who worked tirelessly creating this product and graciously made the many changes recommended by other subject matter experts: Twink Dalton, whose creative juices were never-ending, and John Gosford, whose field experience and technical expertise brought road-ready reality into each case. You two were a dynamic duo. Your shining lights were bright even on the dreariest of days, and your energy and enthusiasm were contagious. A special thank you is also extended to Kim McKenna, who thought it would be fun to write the original study guides and implementation manuals. Your determination to see this project through to its completion, even when the task was arduous and seemed overwhelming, delivered a finished product that is nothing short of genius. We are deeply indebted to each of you and owe you a large replacement supply of midnight oil.

We are also eternally grateful to Jon Cooper, Larry Richmond, and Steve Dralle, who took the challenge to develop this edition of Virtual Patient Encounters for *Paramedic Practice Today: Above and Beyond.* Your tireless efforts have made this study guide and implementation manual the gem it is today.

To paramedic instructors, I hope Virtual Patient Encounters fills in the frustrating gap of trying to prepare students to be critical thinkers and make the right clinical decisions for their patients before these students enter their clinical experiences and the field. Best wishes for great success turning out students who are truly ready for their careers as paramedics.

Finally, thank you to Scott Weaver and Beth LoGiudice for their commitment to produce a dynamic product of the highest quality that will truly prepare paramedic students for a successful career in EMS.

Linda Honeycutt
Executive Editor

Study Guide Reviewers

Jane Bedford, RN, CCEMT-P
Chief Training Officer
Nature Coast EMS
Inverness, Florida

Jon Cooper, NREMT-P
Lieutenant
Baltimore City Fire and EMS Academy
Baltimore, Maryland

John A. DeArmond, NREMT-P
Director
Emergency Management Resources
Half Moon Bay, California

Steven Dralle, BA, LP
Product Marketing Manager
Vidacare
San Antonio, Texas

Dennis Edgerly, EMT-P
Paramedic Education Coordinator
HealthONE EMS
Englewood, Colorado

Janet Fitts, RN, BSN, CEN, TNS, EMT-P
Educational Consultant
Prehospital Emergency Medical Education
Pacific, Missouri

Rudy Garrett, AS, NREMT-P, CCEMT-P
Flight Paramedic
Lifenet Aeromedical Services
Somerset, Kentucky

Mark Goldstein, RN, BSN, EMT-P I/C
EMS Coordinator
William Beaumont Hospital
Royal Oak, Michigan
Adjunct EMS Faculty
Oakland Community College
Auburn Hills, Michigan

John Gosford, BS, EMT-P
Associate Professor and EMS Coordinator
Lake City Community College
Lake City, Florida

Leslie Hernandez, BS, NREMT-P
Advanced Program Director
Bulverde–Spring Branch EMS
Spring Branch, Texas

Scott C. Holliday, BS, EMT-P
Deputy Chief of EMS Training
FDNY
New York, New York

Larry Richmond, AS, NREMT-P, CCEMT-P
EMS Education Manager
Mountain Plains Health Consortium
Ft. Meade, South Dakota

A. Laura Torrez, LP, AAS
EMS Education Coordinator
Methodist Hospital System
Dallas, Texas

Robert Vroman, BS NREMT-P
EMS Instructor
HealthONE EMS
Englewood, Colorado

Getting Started

■ Getting Set Up

SYSTEM REQUIREMENTS

WINDOWS™

- Windows® PC
- Windows XP
- Pentium® processor (or equivalent) @ 1 GHz (2 GHz or greater is recommended)
- 1.5 GB hard disk space
- 512 MB of RAM (1 GB or more is recommended)
- CD-ROM drive
- 800 × 600 screen size
- Thousands of colors
- Soundblaster 16 soundcard compatibility
- Stereo speakers or headphones

MACINTOSH®

Virtual Patient Encounters is not compatible with the Macintosh platform.

INSTALLATION INSTRUCTIONS

WINDOWS™

1. Insert the *Virtual Patient Encounters* CD-ROM.
2. Inserting the CD should automatically bring up the set-up screen if the current product is not already installed.
   a. If the set-up screen does not automatically appear (and *Virtual Patient Encounters* has not been already installed), navigate to the **My Computer** icon on your desktop or in your **Start** menu.

b. Double-click on your CD-ROM drive.

c. If installation does not start at this point:

    (1) Click the **Start** icon on the task bar, and select the **Run** option.

    (2) Type d:\setup.exe (where "d:\" is your CD-ROM drive), and press **OK**.

    (3) Follow the onscreen instructions for installation.

3. Follow the onscreen instructions during the set-up process.

HOW TO LAUNCH *VIRTUAL PATIENT ENCOUNTERS*

WINDOWS™

1. Double-click on the **Virtual Patient Encounters ALS** icon located on your desktop.

2. *(Alternative)* Navigate to the program via the Windows **Start** menu.

SCREEN SETTINGS

For best results, your computer monitor resolution should be set at a minimum of 800 × 600. The number of colors displayed should be set to "thousands or higher" (High Color or 16-bit) or "millions of colors" (True Color or 24-bit).

WINDOWS™

1. From the Start menu, select **Settings**, then **Control Panel**.

2. Double-click on the **Display** icon.

3. Click on the **Settings** tab.

4. Under **Screen Resolution**, use the slider bar to select **800 × 600 pixels**.

5. Access the **Colors** drop-down menu by clicking on the down arrow.

6. Select **High Color (16-bit)** or **True Color (24-bit).**

7. Click on **OK**.

8. You may be asked to verify the setting changes. Click **Yes**.

9. You may be asked to restart your computer to accept the changes. Click **Yes**.

TECHNICAL SUPPORT

Technical support for this product is available between 7:30 AM and 7:00 PM (CST), Monday through Friday. Before calling, be sure your computer meets the recommended system requirements to run this software. Inside the United States and Canada, call 1-800-692-9010. Outside North America, call 1-314-872-8370. You may also fax your questions to 1-314-523-4932, or contact Technical Support through e-mail: technical.support@elsevier.com.

■ Accessing the *Virtual Patient Encounters Online Study Guide* on Evolve

The product you have purchased is part of the Evolve family of online courses and learning resources. Read the following information thoroughly to get started. To access the *Virtual Patient Encounters Online Study Guide* on Evolve, your instructor will provide you with the username and password needed to access the *Virtual Patient Encounters Online Study Guide* on the Evolve Learning System. Once you have received this information, follow these instructions:

1. Go to the Evolve login page (http://evolve.elsevier.com/login).

Trademarks: Windows, Pentium, and America Online are registered trademarks.

2. Enter your username and password in the **Login to My Evolve** area and click the arrow or hit **Enter.**

3. You will be taken to your personalized **My Evolve** page, where the course will be listed in the **My Courses** module.

TECHNICAL REQUIREMENTS

To use the *Virtual Patient Encounters Online Study Guide*, you will need access to a computer that is connected to the Internet and equipped with web browser software that supports frames. For optimal performance, speakers and a high-speed Internet connection are recommended. However, slower dial-up modems (56 K minimum) are acceptable.

WEB BROWSERS

Support web browsers include Microsoft Internet Explorer (IE), version 6.0 or higher; Netscape, version 7.1 or higher; and Mozilla Firefox, version 1.5 or higher.

If you use America Online (AOL) for Web access, you will need AOL, version 4.0 or higher, and IE, version 5.0 or higher. Do not use earlier versions of AOL with earlier versions of IE because you will have difficulty accessing many features.

For best results with AOL:

- Connect to the Internet using AOL, version 4.0 or higher.
- Open a private chat in AOL (this allows the AOL client to remain open without asking whether you wish to disconnect while minimized).
- Minimize AOL.
- Launch a recommended browser.

Whichever browser you use, the browser preferences must be set to enable cookies and JavaScript, and the cache must be set to reload every time.

ENABLE COOKIES

Browser	Steps
Internet Explorer (IE), version 6.0 or higher	1. Select **Tools → Internet Options**. 2. Select **Privacy** tab. 3. Use the slider (slide down) to **Accept All Cookies**. 4. Click **OK**. *OR* 3. Click the **Advanced** button. 4. Click the checkbox next to **Override Automatic Cookie Handling**. 5. Click the **Accept** radio buttons under **First-Party Cookies and Third-Party Cookies**. 6. Click **OK**.
Netscape, version 7.1 or higher	1. Select **Edit → Preferences** 2. Select **Privacy & Security**. 3. Select **Cookies**. 4. Select **Enable All Cookies**.

Browser	Steps
Mozilla Firefox, version 1.5 or higher	1. Select **Tools → Internet Options**. 2. Select the **Privacy** icon. 3. Click to expand **Cookies**. 4. Select **Allow** sites to set cookies. 5. Click **OK**.

ENABLE JAVASCRIPT

Browser	Steps
Internet Explorer (IE), version 6.0 or higher	1. Select **Tools → Internet Options**. 2. Select **Security** tab. 3. Under **Security** level for this zone, set to **Medium** or lower.
Netscape, version 7.1 or higher	1. Select **Edit → Preferences** 2. Select **Advanced**. 3. Select **Scripts & Plugins**. 4. Make sure the **Navigator** box is checked to **Enable JavaScript**. 5. Click **OK**.
Mozilla Firefox, version 1.5 or higher	1. Select **Tools → Options**. 2. Select the **Content** icon. 3. Select **Enable JavaScript**. 4. Click **OK**.

SET CACHE TO ALWAYS RELOAD A PAGE

Browser	Steps
Internet Explorer (IE), version 6.0 or higher	1. Select **Tools → Internet Options**. 2. Select **General** tab. 3. Go to the **Temporary Internet Files**, and click the **Settings** button. 4. Select the radio button for **Every visit to the page**, and click **OK** when complete.
Netscape, version 7.1 or higher	1. Select **Edit → Preferences** 2. Select **Advanced**. 3. Select **Cache**. 4. Select the **Every time I view the page** radio button. 5. Click **OK**.

Browser	Steps
Mozilla Firefox, version 1.5 or higher	1. **Select Tools → Options**. 2. Select the **Privacy** icon. 3. Click to expand **Cache**. 4. Set the value to "**0**" in the **Use up to: ___ MB of disk space for the cache** field. 5. Click **OK**.

PLUG-INS

 Adobe Acrobat Reader—With the free Acrobat Reader software, you can view and print Adobe PDFs. Many Evolve products offer student and instructor manuals, checklists, and more in the PDF format!
Download at: http://www.adobe.com

 Apple QuickTime—Install this software to hear word pronunciations, heart and lung sounds, and many other helpful audio clips in the Evolve Online Courses!
Download at: http://www.apple.com

 Adobe Flash Player—This player will enhance your viewing of many Evolve web pages, as well as educational short- to long-form animation in the Evolve Learning System!
Download at: http://www.adobe.com

 Adobe Shockwave Player—Shockwave is best for viewing the many interactive learning activities in Evolve Online Courses!
Download at: http://www.adobe.com

 Microsoft Word Viewer—With this viewer, Microsoft Word users can share documents with those who do not have Word, and users without Word can open and view Word documents. Many Evolve products have test banks, student and instructor manuals, and other documents available for downloading and viewing on your own computer!
Download at: http://www.microsoft.com

 Microsoft PowerPoint Viewer—View PowerPoint 97, 2000, and 2002 presentations with this viewer, even if you do not have PowerPoint. Many Evolve products have slides available for downloading and viewing on your own computer!
Download at: http://www.microsoft.com

SUPPORT INFORMATION

Live support is available to customers in the United States and Canada from 7:30 AM to 7:00 PM (CST), Monday through Friday, by calling **1-800-401-9962**. You can also send an e-mail to evolve-support@elsevier.com.

In addition, **24/7 support information** is available on the Evolve web site (http://evolve.elsevier.com) including:

- Guided tours
- Tutorials
- Frequently asked questions (FAQs)
- Online copies of course user guides
- And much more!

Orientation to *Virtual Patient Encounters*

Welcome to *Virtual Patient Encounters!*

The course of study to become a paramedic is complex and involves not only a narrow look at a specific topic, but being a paramedic also requires that you have a broad foundation of knowledge from which to pull to enable you to provide effective and safe patient care. Sometimes discrimination among similar choices is required. In the textbooks, patient presentation offers only a clear, one-faceted look at each illness or injury. When reading, patient care may seem similarly straightforward and the path to the correct decisions and interventions may appear very clear. In contrast, real patient situations are often fuzzy, complex, and confusing. This combination of study guide with simulation software is designed to help you bridge the gap between the books and the street and to assist you in "putting it all together." We hope you will reflect on the knowledge from each of the foundation chapters when you evaluate and treat these patients. It is our goal that this course of study will make your transition to the field easier and will give you the confidence to make the right decisions when they matter the most.

BEFORE YOU START

For best results, use the *Virtual Patient Encounters* simulation software as directed by the lessons found in this study guide. Each lesson begins with a reading assignment, usually a single chapter in your textbook. Make sure to read this material before beginning the lesson because you will need to understand the concepts before attempting to answer the questions in the study guide or before you make any patient care decisions in the software. Some lessons also list "relevant" chapters in addition to the reading assignment. These *summative* lessons will require a broad understanding of many concepts from different topic areas before being attempted. We highly recommend that you read all of these relevant chapters in addition to the reading assignment before attempting the summative lessons.

The following icons are used throughout the study guide to help you quickly identify particular activities and assignments:

Reading Assignment—Tells you which textbook chapter(s) you should read before starting each lesson.

Writing Activity—Certain activities focus on written responses such as filling out forms or completing documentation.

 CD-ROM Activity—Marks the beginning of an activity that uses the *Virtual Patient Encounters* simulation software.

 Reference—Indicates questions and activities that require you to consult your textbook.

Time—Indicates the approximate amount of time needed to complete the exercise.

Each lesson in the study guide provides specific directions that explain what to do in the software to prepare for each exercise. These directions are always bulleted and are always indicated by an arrow (→) in the left margin. Do no more or no less than what the directions indicate. For example, many lessons require that you watch only a video before answering the study guide questions, whereas others will direct you to also perform your initial assessment in the software. Summative lessons will direct you to care for the patient from beginning to end as best you can, based on what you have learned from the textbook and in class.

Although the study guide lessons provide specific directions as to what to do in the software, when it comes to caring for the patients (e.g., performing assessments and interventions), you will need to understand what all the buttons do. The following orientation will explain the entire software interface and how you can treat each of the 15 cases.

HOW TO LOG IN

To open the *Virtual Patient Encounters* simulation program, you can either double click the *Virtual Patient Encounters ALS* icon that should appear on your computer desktop after you have installed the software, or you can click on **Start**, then **Programs**, then **Virtual Patient Encounters**, then **Virtual Patient Encounters ALS**. Once the program begins, you will see an anti-piracy warning and a video montage before the log-on screen appears (shown below). If you wish to skip the video montage, click on the **Skip Intro** button at the bottom of the screen.

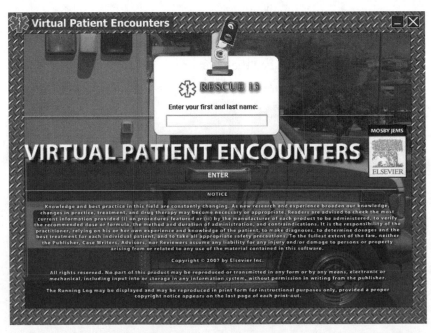

Type your first and last names into the name tag pictured, and click **Enter.** This will take you to a list of all 15 cases in this program (shown in the first screen on the following page).

Once you click on a patient, you can listen to the dispatch report, which will also appear as text in the panel on the right side of the screen. (If you do not want to hear the dispatch audio, you can click on the **MUTE** icon.) After you have listened to and read the dispatch information, you can then click **START** to respond to the case. (An **EXIT** button also appears on this screen if you want to close the entire program.)

Once you select a case, your initial approach to the scene and patient will play in a video. All the videos include an overview of the area from the perspective of the ambulance (shown below) to enable you to think about staging considerations and scene safety.

On approaching the patient, you will have an opportunity to perform the scene size-up, form an initial visual impression of the patient, and listen to information provided by conscious patients and any first responders, family members, or bystanders on the scene. Be aware that

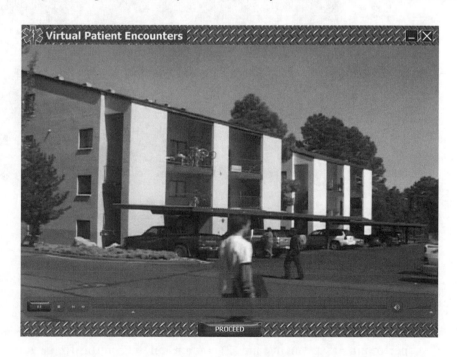

some videos intentionally deviate from "best practice" to give you a chance to critique how things were handled. In addition, interventions, such as spinal immobilization, which would have been performed immediately in some cases, were not shown in the video to give you the opportunity to make all the decisions about patient care once the video concludes.

The video controls are similar to those found in many popular media players. Here is what each one does:

II (Pause)—Pauses or "freezes" the video on the current frame.

▶ **PLAY**—Resumes playing the video from the point where it has been paused or from the beginning if the video has been stopped.

■ **STOP**—Stops the video entirely. To restart the video, you must click **PLAY** (▶).

◀◀ **REWIND**—Restarts the video from the beginning.

▶▶ **FORWARD**—Jumps several frames forward in the video.

Two slider bars are also provided. The long slider bar across most of the width of the screen allows you to scroll back and forth to any point in the video. Simply double click and hold the triangle (▲), then drag it to the left to go to an earlier moment or to the right to go to a later moment. The short slider bar on the far right controls the volume of the video's audio. A mute button between the two slider bars can be clicked to turn off the audio altogether.

When the video reaches the end, it automatically will forward you to the patient care interface, which is described below. If you want to skip the video altogether and go directly to the patient care interface, you can click on the **PROCEED** button at the bottom of the video screen.

PATIENT CARE INTERFACE

The patient care interface consists of three panels: (1) Patient Care Panel, (2) Patient Visual Panel, and (3) Running Log as described in the following text.

Patient Care Panel

The Patient Care Panel runs along the left side of the screen and consists primarily of two distinct areas (shown at the top of the following page): (1) contains all the controls for performing assessments and (2) contains all the controls for performing interventions.

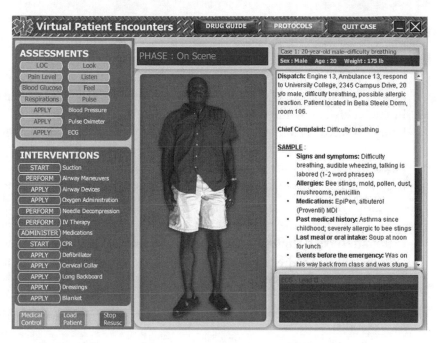

Assessment Controls

The assessment controls allow you to gather information on each patient so you can decide which interventions would be appropriate to care for him or her. These control buttons allow you to perform your patient assessments. Each button is described individually.

LOC (Level of Consciousness)—Click the **LOC** button to reveal the patient's current level of consciousness in the running log on the right side of the screen. In some cases the patient's orientation will be below the level of consciousness if it is pertinent to the case. Be aware that the patient's level of consciousness may change, depending on what interventions you perform. For instance, administering a sedative may decrease the patient's level of consciousness.

Pain Level—Click the **Pain Level** button to reveal the patient's current pain level on the 1-to-10 scale. The patient's pain level can increase or decrease, depending on your treatment; for example, administering a narcotic to a patient with a high pain level may decrease his or her level of pain.

Blood Glucose—Click the **Blood Glucose** button to reveal the patient's current blood glucose reading. Treatments such as administering 50% dextrose could affect this reading.

Respirations—Click the **Respirations** button to reveal the patient's current respiratory rate and quality. The respiration rate and quality can also be affected by your patient care decisions. For example, the patient's respiratory rate will slow after administering midazolam.

Pulse—Click the **Pulse** button to reveal the patient's current pulse rate, regularity, and strength. Your patient care decisions can affect these three measurements. For example, administering atropine sulfate will slow the patient's heart rate.

Blood Pressure—Click the **APPLY** button for blood pressure to place a blood pressure cuff on the patient and to receive your first reading. Once the cuff is on the patient, you only need to click the **READ** button that appears to the right for subsequent readings. If you want to remove the blood pressure cuff, you can click the **REMOVE** button that replaces the **APPLY** button. Interventions such as dopamine administration can affect blood pressure.

Pulse Oximeter—Click the **APPLY** button for pulse oximeter to place a finger clip on the patient and to receive your first oxygen saturation (SaO_2) reading. Once the clip is on the patient, you only need to click the **READ** button that appears to the right for subsequent readings. If you want to remove the finger clip, you can click the **REMOVE** button that replaces the **APPLY** button. Interventions such as administering oxygen to the patient in respiratory distress can affect SaO_2 readings.

ECG—Click the **APPLY** button next to the ECG button to place leads on the patient and display a dynamic ECG tracing on the monitor in the lower right corner of the screen, immediately below the running log. Note that this ECG is a 3-lead ECG and that lead II is being displayed. Twelve-lead ECGs for several cases are included in the relevant study guide lessons for your evaluation. If you want to remove the ECG, you can click the **REMOVE** button that replaces the **APPLY** button. Make sure to keep your eyes on the ECG tracing because it can change unexpectedly or in response to your treatment decisions.

Look—Click the **Look** button to open a "wizard" that allows you to receive visual information about the patient's head and neck, chest and abdomen, upper extremities, lower extremities, back, and genitalia. Simply click on the body area you want to know about, and then click **ASSESS**. (Click **CANCEL** if you want to exit the wizard.) The following information is displayed in the running log for each body area:

Head and Neck
- Pupil size[*]
- Pupil reactivity[*]
- Skin color[*]
- Mouth[*]
- Nose[*]
- Other observations
- DCAP-BTLS

Chest and Abdomen
- Check excursion[*]
- Skin color[*]
- Other observations
- DCAP-BTLS

Upper Extremities
- Skin color[*]
- Other observations
- DCAP-BTLS

Lower Extremities
- Skin color[*]
- Other observations
- DCAP-BTLS

Back
- Skin color[*]
- Other observations
- DCAP-BTLS

Genitalia
- Other observations
- DCAP-BTLS

[*]This may change in response to your treatment decisions; do not forget to reassess often.

Listen—Click the **Listen** button to open a wizard that allows you to receive aural information about the patient's heart and lungs. Simply click on the organ you want to know about, and then click **ASSESS**. (Click **CANCEL** if you want to exit the wizard.) The following information is displayed in the running log for each:

Heart
- Heart rate*
- Heart regularity*

Lungs
- Left lung sounds*
- Right lung sounds*

Feel—Click the **Feel** button to open a wizard that allows you to receive tactile information about the patient's head and neck, chest and abdomen, upper extremities, lower extremities, and back. Simply click on the body area you want to know about and then click **ASSESS**. (Click **CANCEL** if you want to exit the wizard.) The following information is displayed in the running log for each body area:

Head and Neck
- Skin temperature*
- Skin moisture*
- Other observations
- DCAP-BTLS

Chest and Abdomen
- Skin temperature*
- Skin moisture*
- Other observations
- DCAP-BTLS

Upper Extremities
- Skin temperature*
- Skin moisture*
- Other observations
- DCAP-BTLS

Lower Extremities
- Skin temperature*
- Skin moisture*
- Other observations
- DCAP-BTLS

Back
- Skin temperature*
- Skin moisture*
- Other observations
- DCAP-BTLS

*This may change in response to your treatment decisions; do not forget to reassess often.

Intervention Controls

The intervention buttons will allow you to treat each patient in accordance with what you have learned in your textbook and in class, as well as what you think are the issues with each patient based on information you have gathered from the opening video, the patient's history, and any assessments you have performed. Each intervention that you perform may cause realistic changes in the patient, which you can determine by conducting ongoing assessments. Each intervention button is described individually below.

Suction—Click **START** to clear the patient's airway. Click **STOP** to end suctioning.

Airway Maneuvers—Click **PERFORM** to open a wizard that will allow you to choose to perform an abdominal thrust, a head-tilt/chin-lift, or a jaw thrust. Simply click on the maneuver you would like to perform.

Airway Devices—Click **APPLY** to open a wizard that will allow you to choose from the following airway devices:

- Oropharyngeal airway
- Nasopharyngeal airway
- Endotracheal tube
- Laryngeal mask
- Cricothyrotomy
- Combitube

If you select the endotracheal tube, you will be prompted to select multiple methods for confirming the correct tube placement. Click **REMOVE** to remove the airway device currently in use.

Oxygen Administration—Click **APPLY** to open a wizard that will allow you select from the following types of oxygen and ventilation devices:

- Nasal cannula
- Simple face mask
- Partial rebreather mask
- Nonrebreather mask
- Bag-mask at 12 breaths/min
- Bag-mask at 20 breaths/min

Once you select one of the above devices, you will be prompted to select an oxygen flow rate. Click **REMOVE** to remove the type of oxygen or ventilation device currently in use.

Needle Decompression—Click **PERFORM** to open a wizard that will allow you to select a needle gauge before performing needle decompression. Because needle decompression is an intervention that cannot be undone, the program will not permit you to perform this intervention on any patient for whom it would be inappropriate.

IV Therapy—Click **PERFORM** to open a wizard that will allow you to start an intravenous (IV) or intraosseous line for medication administration or fluid therapy.

Five steps to this wizard are listed as follows:

1. Select whether you want to start a left or right peripheral IV or get intraosseous access (shown at the top of the following page). Click **NEXT** after you have made your choice (or **CANCEL** to close the wizard altogether).
2. Select which type of fluid you want to infuse. Click **NEXT** after you have made your choice (or **BACK** to return to the previous step or **CANCEL** to close the wizard altogether).

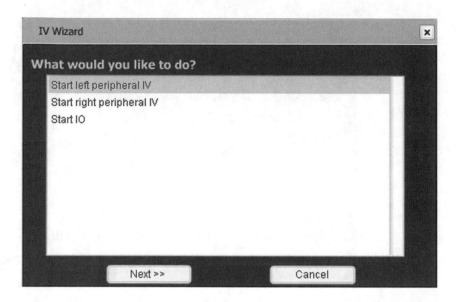

3. Select the rate of infusion you want—select either TKO (to keep open) to provide a route for administering medications or wide open for fluid replacement therapy. Wide open can also be used to administer medications intravenously in addition to fluid therapy. Click **NEXT** after you have made your choice (or **BACK** to return to the previous step or **CANCEL** to close the wizard altogether).

4. If you chose TKO on the third step, the next step allows you to select your catheter size and tubing. If you chose Wide Open on the third step, you have to select your fluid amount before you select your catheter size and tubing. Always click **NEXT** to advance to the next step, **BACK** to return to the previous step, or **CANCEL** to close the wizard altogether.

5. The last step allows you to confirm all your selections before committing to them. Read over what you selected; if your selections are what you want, then click **DONE**. If you want to make modifications, click **BACK** to return to the step where you want to make changes. Make your changes, and click **NEXT** until you get back to the confirmation step. As always, clicking the **CANCEL** button will close the wizard without any effect on the patient.

Once you have started an IV or intraosseous line, you can reopen the IV Therapy Wizard again and again by clicking **PERFORM**. When you reopen the wizard, you will see a slightly different set of options at the first step. You can choose one of the following:

1. Start another line,

2. Remove a line that you have already started, or

3. Administer additional fluids to any of the lines you already started.

   Use the **NEXT, BACK**, and **DONE** buttons to make and confirm your selections.

   You will also notice that a **FLUSH** button appears in the panel to the right once you have started a line. You can click on this button and flush any of the lines that you have already started.

   Medications—Click **ADMINISTER** to open a wizard that allows you to administer medications to the patient.

   The wizard has four steps:

1. Select the medication you want to administer from the alphabetical list of generic drug names displayed (see figure on the following page). You can review the list of medications

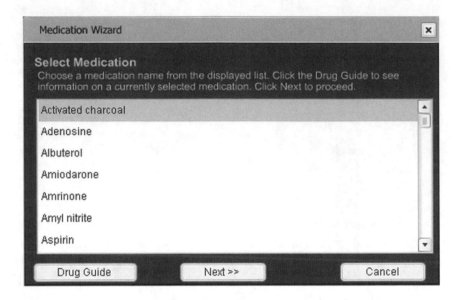

using the scroll bar on the right side of the wizard. If you want to look up more information about a drug, click the **Drug Guide** button. This button will open a searchable resource that will be described in greater detail later in this orientation session. Highlight the medication you want to administer by clicking on its name, and then click **NEXT**. (Click **CANCEL** to exit the wizard altogether.)

2. Select the route you want to use to administer the drug you selected in the first step. Again, you can review the list of routes using the scroll bar on the right. (Note that the IV and intraosseous routes will not appear on this list unless you have already started them using the IV Therapy Wizard as previously described. If you need to administer a drug using one of these routes, click **CANCEL** to close the medication wizard and then open the IV Therapy Wizard to start a line first. Then you can reopen the medication wizard, and you will now find the route listed at the second step.) Highlight the route you want to use, and then click **NEXT**. (Click **CANCEL** to exit the wizard altogether.) If you select an incorrect route for the drug you selected at the first step, you will receive a message to that effect and be instructed to click **BACK** and make a different route selection. Be aware that your incorrect route selection will be recorded on the running log, so make your selections carefully.

3. Select the dose you want to administer of the drug you selected in the first step. Be aware that each dose may have a different effect on the patient. Highlight the dose you want to administer, and then click **NEXT**. (Click **CANCEL** to exit the wizard altogether.)

4. The last step allows you to confirm all your selections before committing to them. Read over what you selected; if all selections are what you want, then click **FINISH**. If you want to make modifications, click **BACK** to return to the step where you want to make changes. Make your changes, and click **NEXT** until you get back to the confirmation step. As always, **CANCEL** will close the wizard without any effect on the patient. Note that if you select the IV or intraosseous route at the second step, you will have to select whether you want to inject the medication as an IV push or IV infusion before you can confirm your selections. You must select an IV type that is compatible with the medication and dose you selected earlier to proceed. If you make the wrong selection, your mistake will be recorded in the running log.

CPR—Click **START** to begin performing cardiopulmonary resuscitation (CPR) on the patient. Click **STOP** to stop CPR.

Defibrillator—Click **APPLY** to place defibrillator pads on the patient. Click **REMOVE** to remove the pads. To defibrillate the patient, click on the **PACE/SHOCK** button that appears in the panel to the right. This selection will open a wizard; you must first select whether you want to start pacing or to shock the patient in either sync or unsync mode. If you start pacing the patient, you have to reopen this wizard to stop pacing. If you choose to shock the patient in either sync or unsync mode, you will then be prompted to select an energy level. When you click on an energy level, the shock will be delivered to the patient. You can also click **BACK** to return to the initial screen or **CANCEL** to close the wizard without any effects on the patient.

IMPORTANT: Be aware that the defibrillator simulated in the software is intended to be used as a monophasic machine. A monophasic defibrillator was simulated instead of a biphasic machine because recommended energy levels are consistent from manufacturer to manufacturer, whereas energy levels for biphasic machines currently vary, depending on the make of the machine. Although biphasic defibrillators have become common, monophasic machines are still in use and may be encountered both in the classroom and in the field. Keep this in mind when selecting which energy level to administer when using the defibrillator.

Cervical Collar—Click **APPLY** to place a cervical collar on the patient. Click **REMOVE** to remove it.

Long Backboard—Click **APPLY** to place the patient on a long backboard. Click **REMOVE** to remove it.

Dressings—Click **APPLY** to place dressings on any wounds the patient may have. (Nothing will happen if the patient does not have wounds.) Click **REMOVE** to remove the dressings.

Blanket—Click **APPLY** to place a blanket on the patient. Click **REMOVE** to remove the blanket.

"Other" Buttons

Three additional buttons below the intervention controls level are available for use during patient care:

Medical Control—Click the **Medical Control** button if you want to contact medical control. In this program you can contact medical control to request additional orders or to request permission to stop resuscitation. Consult medical control if you are having trouble figuring out which protocol(s) to follow for a particular case. They will eventually point you in the right direction. They will give you permission to stop resuscitation only if resuscitating the patient is not possible.

Stop Resusc—If medical control gives you permission to stop resuscitation, you may click the **Stop Rescusc** button. If you click the **Stop Resusc** button, you will be asked to confirm your decision. If you click *yes* to confirm, stopping resuscitation will be recorded in your log. Keep in mind that if you stop resuscitation without requesting permission from medical control or if permission was denied, all of this will be recorded in your log for your instructor to evaluate.

Load/Unload Patient—When you first enter the patient care interface, you are considered to be "on scene." While on scene this button will display as **Load Patient**. Click this button when you believe transporting the patient is most appropriate. Your decision to load will be recorded in the running log in the context of all your assessments and interventions. Once you have loaded the patient, you are considered to be in transit and this button changes to display as **Unload Patient**.

You may have noticed that time is not counted in this program. Although this is a luxury you will not have in real life, removing the time element allows you to think about your decisions before you make them, rather than simply trying to "beat the clock," particularly because assessments and interventions are not done in real time. *Virtual Patient Encounters* is not intended to be used as a game.

Although the study guide may pose situations in which you have limited time in transit and asks questions about how you would adjust your treatment, in the software program you can continue performing interventions and assessments while in transit for as long as you believe you can make a difference. Once there is nothing more you can do besides provide support and monitor your patient, then you can click **UNLOAD PATIENT**.

Patient Visual Panel

The panel in the middle of the interface displays the patient in the supine position from a top-down perspective (shown below).

As you perform your assessments and interventions, the equipment you use appears on the patient in this panel. For example, when you click **APPLY Blood Pressure**, a blood pressure cuff will appear on the patient's arm; and when you click **APPLY Oxygen Administration** and select a nonrebreather mask, an image of a nonrebreather mask will appear on the patient; and so on. The patient visual panel is intended to give you a visual indication of what equipment is currently in use on the patient. The equipment images are representative of real equipment but may not always appear exactly as they would in real life; for example, when a long backboard is used, the patient would be secured to it with straps and a head immobilization device.

When you start CPR using the intervention buttons, you will see a pair of hands repeatedly compressing the patient's chest. These hands will give you a visual indication that CPR is in progress. When you stop CPR, the hands will disappear.

The patient is supine to best display the equipment that is in use. This position does not represent the position in which the patient is found nor does it necessarily represent the position in which you would place the patient to perform proper care. Questions about positioning of each of the patients will be found in the study guide lessons.

Above the patient visual, a display indicates whether you are "On Scene" or "In Transit."

Running Log

The running log is seen on the right side of the interface (shown below).

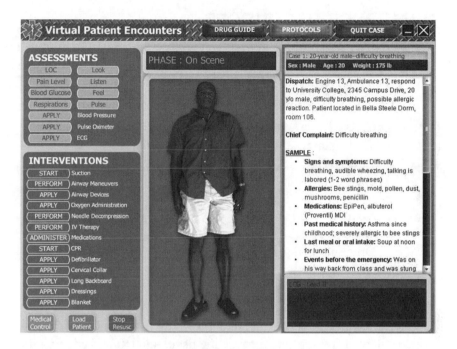

When you first enter the patient care interface after watching the video, the log will display the initial dispatch that you heard, as well as the patient's chief complaint and history in SAMPLE/OPQRST format. You should read this information before making any assessment or intervention decisions because doing so will provide a more complete picture than the video alone.

Once you begin making assessments, the data and observations appear in the running log in the order that you perform the assessments below the **Now On Scene** heading. This running log lets you know what is happening with the patient and, by reassessing, what is changing about the patient.

All interventions that you perform are also recorded in the running log. Interventions are always listed in italics to distinguish them from assessments. All the choices you make within the steps of the intervention wizards are recorded on the log; for example, when administering medications, the dose and the route are recorded in addition to the drug name.

Certain messages appear in the log in red type, either to notify you that something drastic has changed about your patient or to let you know that something you tried to do was not possible and why. For example, if your patient becomes unconscious while you are treating him or her, you may receive the message, "Your patient's condition has changed. You need to reassess," or "Patient is exhibiting seizure activity." If you were to try to defibrillate while performing CPR, you would receive a message such as, "Unable to perform defibrillator unsync shock, you are still doing CPR." Once you stop CPR, you can defibrillate.

As your running log fills up with more and more information, you can use the scroll bar on the right to scroll up and down, perhaps to compare assessment data before and after a particular intervention.

Note that the case number and complaint, as well as the patient's gender, age, and weight, are listed for your information across the top of the running log.

Below the running log, an ECG display appears. As mentioned earlier, this display depicts lead II of a three-lead ECG.

REFERENCE RESOURCES

Across the top of the interface, you will see a blue button marked **DRUG GUIDE** and a yellow button labeled **PROTOCOLS**, which can be used as reference resources.

Clicking **DRUG GUIDE** will open a new window in which you can review the following information about medications from the Emergency Drug Index in your textbook:

- Class
- Trade names
- Description
- Onset and duration
- Indications
- Contraindications
- Adverse reactions
- Drug interactions
- How supplied
- Dosage and administration
- Special considerations

You can look up a drug either by typing its generic name in the search field at the top of the window or by scrolling through the list on the left and clicking directly on its name. To close the drug guide window, click on the **X** in the upper right corner.

Clicking **PROTOCOLS** opens a different window that displays a menu of 23 protocols that were developed in accordance with your textbook and the *1998 National Standard Curriculum for the EMT-Paramedic*. One or more of these protocols will be appropriate for each of the 15 cases found in this program. Simply click on the name of the protocol you want to open. Note that each protocol is divided into sections by scope of practice. Although the protocols will not tell you exactly what to do, keep in mind that they should put you on the right track if you have selected protocols that are relevant to the patient you are treating.

To return to the listing of protocols, click on **Return to List**. To close the protocols window, click on the **X** in the upper right corner.

SUMMARY MENU

Three ways are provided to navigate to the summary menu, two of which you already know about; that is, by clicking **Unload Patient** while in transit or by clicking **Stop Resusc** after you have been given permission to do so by medical control. The third way is by clicking the red **QUIT CASE** button to the right of the **PROTOCOLS** button. Use this button to leave a case when you want to skip it or to switch to another case. Many study guide lessons may only require you to watch the video and read the history before answering the questions, in which case you will be directed to simply quit the case.

The summary menu itself offers four choices as described below:

LOG—Click the **Log** button to view, save, or print the log from the case you just completed. The information that was recorded in the running log during patient care is now displayed full screen for you to review easily (shown below).

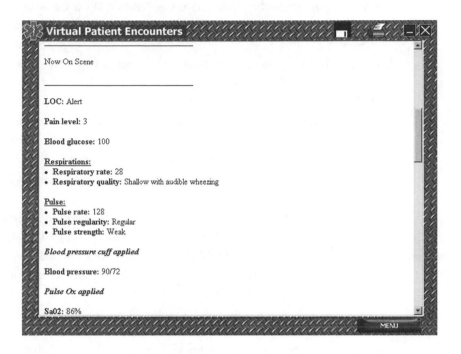

All of the summative lessons will instruct you to review the log of your patient care while answering questions in the study guide. Click the icon of the floppy disk in the upper right corner to save your log as a rich text file, or click the icon of a printer to print out a hard copy. Be prepared for your instructor to ask you to submit your logs for his or her evaluation. Click **MENU** in the lower right corner to return to the summary menu.

RESTART—Click the **Restart** button to return to the patient selection screen. Be aware that unless you printed or saved a copy of your log from the case you just completed, a record of what you did will not be available to retrieve.

CREDITS—Click the **Credits** button to display a listing of all the people and organizations that contributed to the development of the simulation software. Click **RETURN TO MENU** to return to the summary menu.

EXIT—Click the **Exit** button to close the entire *Virtual Patient Encounters* program. As with clicking **RESTART**, be aware that unless you printed or saved a copy of your log from the case you just completed, no record of what you did will be available to retrieve.

TIPS FOR USING *VIRTUAL PATIENT ENCOUNTERS*

Last, the following tips will improve your experience with *Virtual Patient Encounters* and can enhance your knowledge and prepare you for facing the uncertainty of the streets.

1. Always read the assigned chapter(s) before attempting the study guide lessons.

2. Keep your textbook handy as a reference while you work through the lessons.

3. Take your time—things in the program are not happening in real time. Reflect on your next action before you perform it.

4. Be sure to think about the appropriate sequence of actions. In real life, many assessments and interventions will happen simultaneously. When working in this program, you have to perform things one step at a time. For example, if you elect to intubate, you will have to stop bag-mask ventilation first.

5. Do not assume that others are performing certain skills or assessments as they would on a real call. You must specifically identify each assessment and intervention to be performed on the call.

6. Use the running log to review and reflect on what you have done so you can choose your next intervention or assessment.

7. Watch for the key messages (in red type) that may appear in the running log to indicate that the patient's condition has changed drastically. Failure to see one of these messages can lead you down the wrong path.

8. Just as you would in real life, reassess often, particularly after any significant intervention.

9. Because you do not interact with a live patient, you will not have benefit of the information and clues that you would normally have. Things such as how the patient feels (except for pain scale), his or her body language, and additional environmental clues will not be available. Simply use the information that you have and make the best judgments you can, based on the information you are given.

10. When you use the software program, follow the bulleted directions provided in the lessons and answer the relevant questions.

11. In some cases, you may think that an intervention or drug dose is appropriate but not available. Make the best choice available. This will prepare you for the "real world" of EMS where everything you need is also not available. Sometimes you have to improvise and do the best you can with what you have. The ability to make the most with the least is often what makes a great paramedic.

12. As previously mentioned, the protocols follow the guidelines in your textbook—sometimes these will vary from your local protocols. Discuss any variations and the reasons for them with your instructor.

13. The exact nature of illness or injury may not be perfectly clear in all cases. In other cases, you may have a pretty clear clinical impression, but you might not have any interventions that can correct the patient's problem. This scenario also mirrors real EMS practice. Simply perform the best interventions at your disposal and transport the patient when appropriate. Limitations in the prehospital setting will always occur.

We hope that *Virtual Patient Encounters* will be just one more tool to build your knowledge and improve your critical thinking ability as you move toward your goal to becoming a paramedic. Best wishes and good luck!

EMS Safety and Well-Being of the Paramedic

 Reading Assignment: Read Chapter 1, EMS Safety and Well-Being of the Paramedic, in *Paramedic Practice Today: Above and Beyond.*

Case 12: 57-year-old male—man down

Case 1: 20-year-old male—difficulty breathing

Case 3: 7-year-old female—seizure

Objectives:

On completion of this lesson, the student will be able to perform the following:

- Discuss the risk factors and warning signs of cardiovascular disease.
- Discuss proper lifting techniques and safety factors related to lifting and moving patients during emergency and nonemergency situations.
- Discuss the steps that should be taken to protect yourself from airborne and blood-borne pathogens, as well as other adverse conditions and situations.
- Discuss actions that reduce infectious disease exposure as related to field scenarios.
- Discuss how paramedics deal with stressed patients, families, death, and dying.

EXERCISE 1

 CD-ROM Activity

 Time: 10 minutes

→
- Sign into the software by entering your name in the name tag and clicking **Enter.**
- Choose the case by clicking on *Case 12: 57-year-old male—man down.*
- Listen to the dispatch, or read it in the right panel (or both).
- Click **Start** and watch the entire video. Once the video has concluded, you are "on scene."

1. What lifting techniques did you observe the paramedics demonstrate that should reduce the risk of back injury on the job?

2. How can paramedics reduce their susceptibility to heat-related illness while on the job?

3. What measures were the paramedics using to reduce their risk of exposure to blood or bloody bodily fluids? Discuss the reasons you believe these measures are adequate or the reasons they are not.

→
- Click **Quit Case,** and you will be taken to the summary menu.

EXERCISE 2

 CD-ROM Activity

 Time: 10 minutes

- Click **Restart** from the summary menu.
- Choose the case by clicking on *Case 1: 20-year-old male—difficulty breathing.*
- Listen to the dispatch, or read it in the right panel (or both).
- Click **Start** and watch the entire video. Once the video has concluded, you are "on scene."

4. List measures you can take to minimize the risk of injury to the crew or the patient if the patient is conscious but cannot walk down the stairs.

5. What individual characteristics about the paramedics did you note that might reduce the patient's risk of injury or illness?

6. If the paramedics worked several consecutive shifts and were severely sleep deprived, how could that condition influence their performance on this call?

7. What measures, aside from gloves and other standard precautions, should the paramedics take to reduce their risk of getting or spreading infectious disease?

   a. Preventative measures to take while on the job:

   b. Preventive measures to take that protect them on every call:

 • Click **Quit Case,** and you will be taken to the summary menu.
   • Click **Exit** to close the program, or **Restart** to continue with another lesson.

EXERCISE 3

 CD-ROM Activity

 Time: 10 minutes

 • Click **Restart** from the summary menu.
   • Choose the case by clicking on *Case 3: 7-year-old female—seizure.*
   • Listen to the dispatch, or read it in the right panel (or both).
   • Click **Start** and watch the entire video. Once the video has concluded, you are "on scene."

8. Once the paramedics enter the home, the adult male becomes aggressive. Did the paramedics handle the situation appropriately? Why or why not?

9. The paramedics have begun to treat the patient in this case when the adult male becomes aggressive. Should the paramedics leave the patient to ensure their safety? How would the paramedics safeguard themselves and the patient?

→ • Click **Quit Case,** and you will be taken to the summary menu.
  • Click **Exit** to close the program, or **Restart** to continue with another lesson.

Paramedic Roles and Responsibilities

Reading Assignment: Read Chapter 2, Paramedic Roles and Responsibilities, in *Paramedic Practice Today: Above and Beyond*.

Case 10: 25-year-old female—abdominal pain

Case 9: 22-year-old female—assault

Objectives:

On completion of this lesson, the student will be able to perform the following:

- Describe how the attributes of the paramedic professional are demonstrated during patient care activities.

EXERCISE 1

  CD-ROM Activity

 Time: 15 minutes

- Sign into the software by entering your name in the name tag and clicking **Enter.**
- Choose the case by clicking on *Case 10: 25-year-old female—abdominal pain.*
- Listen to the dispatch, or read it in the right panel (or both).
- Click **Start** and watch the entire video. Once the video has concluded, you are "on scene."
- Read the history log on the right side of the screen.

1. Describe specific behaviors you observed of the paramedics on this call that demonstrate the attributes of the professional paramedic. If the attribute is not seen on this call, then write *not observed.*

Attribute	Specific Behavior Observed on This Call
Integrity	
Empathy	

Attribute	Specific Behavior Observed on This Call
Self-motivation	
Appearance and personal hygiene	
Self-confidence	
Communications	

Attribute	Specific Behavior Observed on This Call
Time management	
Teamwork and diplomacy	
Respect	
Patient advocacy	

Attribute	Specific Behavior Observed on This Call
Careful delivery of service	

2. On this case, why will it be important for the paramedic to have a good working knowledge of hospital designation and categorization?

3. Describe what type of online or offline medical direction the paramedics may need on this call.

   a. Online medical direction:

   b. Offline medical direction:

 • Click **Quit Case,** and you will be taken to the summary menu.
• Click **Exit** to close the program, or **Restart** to continue with another lesson.

EXERCISE 2

 CD-ROM Activity

 Time: 15 minutes

- Click **Restart** from the summary menu.
- Choose the case by clicking on *Case 9: 22-year-old female—assault.*
- Listen to the dispatch, or read it in the right panel (or both).
- Click **Start** and watch the entire video. Once the video has concluded, you are "on scene."
- Read the history log on the right side of the screen.

4. Describe why each of these professional attributes is important on this call. Then, describe whether you observed them in the brief time you had to observe the paramedics on the call.

Attribute	Importance? Observed on This Call?
Integrity	
Empathy	

Attribute	Importance? Observed on This Call?
Self-motivation	
Appearance and personal hygiene	
Self-confidence	
Communications	

Attribute	Importance? Observed on This Call?
Time management	
Teamwork and diplomacy	
Respect	
Patient advocacy	
Careful delivery of service	

- Click **Quit Case,** and you will be taken to the summary menu.
- Click **Exit** to close the program, or **Restart** to continue with another lesson.

Illness and Injury Prevention

Reading Assignment: Read Chapter 3, Illness and Injury Prevention, in *Paramedic Practice Today: Above and Beyond*.

Case 7: 8-year-old male—submersion

Case 2: 56-year-old female—fell

Objectives:

On completion of this lesson, the student will be able to perform the following:

- Apply Haddon's matrix to selected cases to identify factors that contribute to injury.
- Relate injury prevention principles to selected cases.
- Identify resources available to develop an injury prevention program.

EXERCISE 1

 CD-ROM Activity

 Time: 15 minutes

- Sign into the software by entering your name in the name tag and clicking **Enter.**
- Choose the case by clicking on *Case 7: 8-year-old male—submersion.*
- Listen to the dispatch, or read it in the right panel (or both).
- Click **Start** and watch the entire video. Once the video has concluded, you are "on scene."
- Read the history log on the right side of the screen.

1. Complete the following table to relate the components of Haddon's matrix to this call.

Phase	Host	Agent	Environment
Pre-event			

2. Discuss how the six *E*'s of injury prevention could be applied to prevent children from drowning.

   a. Education:

   b. Enforcement:

   c. Engineering:

    d. Environment:

    e. EMS:

    f. Economic incentives:

3. If the child in this case survives the injury, predict costs (not in actual dollars) that will be associated with this injury.

4. Is there a teachable moment in this case?

→ • Click **Quit Case,** and you will be taken to the summary menu.
   • Click **Exit** to close the program, or **Restart** to continue with another lesson.

EXERCISE 2

 CD-ROM Activity

 Time: 15 minutes

- Click **Restart** from the summary menu.
- Choose the case by clicking on *Case 2: 56-year-old female—fell.*
- Listen to the dispatch, or read it in the right panel (or both).
- Click **Start** and watch the entire video. Once the video has concluded, you are "on scene."
- Read the history log on the right side of the screen.

5. What pre-event factors contribute to fall-related injuries in older adults?

Host	Agent	Environment

- Answer the following questions that relate to developing a fall-prevention program in your community.

6. What resources would you use to find out the incidence and cost of older adult, fall-related injuries in your community?

7. How will you determine how many older adults live in your community?

8. Where can you ask for money to help fund your program?

9. You decide to develop a written flyer as part of your injury-prevention program. How can you make sure that it will be effective and understood by your intended audience?

10. How can you measure the effectiveness of your program?

 • Click **Quit Case** and you will be taken to the summary menu.
• Click **Exit** to close the program, or **Restart** to continue with another lesson.

Legal and Regulatory Issues

✎ **Reading Assignment:** Read Chapter 4, Legal and Regulatory Issues, in *Paramedic Practice Today: Above and Beyond*.

Case 3: 7-year-old female—seizure

Case 4: 64-year-old male—unknown medical

Case 9: 22-year-old female—assault

Objectives:

On completion of this lesson, the student will be able to perform the following:

- Differentiate between legal and ethical responsibilities.
- Describe the four elements that must be present to prove negligence.
- Determine whether the four components of negligence are present in the scenario in which a patient is injured.
- Identify patient care behaviors that would protect the paramedic from claims of negligence.
- Describe the differences among expressed, informed, implied, and involuntary consent.
- Identify the steps to take if a patient refuses care.

EXERCISE 1

 CD-ROM Activity

 Time: 15 minutes

- Click **Restart** from the summary menu.
- Choose the case by clicking on *Case 3: 7-year-old female—seizure.*
- Listen to the dispatch, or read it in the right panel (or both).
- Click **Start** and watch the entire video. Once the video has concluded, you are "on scene."

1. Which of the parents is giving consent for the treatment of Jenny? How does the parent go about giving consent? Based on the video, is the treatment informed?

2. Why should consent not be obtained from Jenny's father? How should the paramedics proceed if the father is the only parent present?

3. Jenny's mother suddenly agrees with her husband's wish and asks the paramedics to leave. How should the paramedics address the sudden change of heart?

4. During the care of Jenny, her father comes out of his room and assaults Jenny's mother and sibling. How should the paramedics react to this occurrence?

5. Where can the paramedics find the standard of care for Jenny in this scenario? What care should be delivered to Jenny according to the standard of care?

6. Jenny has an adverse reaction to a medication administered during treatment. Jenny's mother reported an allergy only to penicillin. The reaction results in a lengthy hospital stay and many months of rehabilitation for Jenny. Explain how the paramedics can be responsible for this, even though they were doing "the right thing."

- Click **Quit Case** and you will be taken to the summary menu.
- Click **Exit** to close the program, or **Restart** to continue with another lesson.

EXERCISE 2

 CD-ROM Activity

 Time: 15 minutes

- Click **Restart** from the summary menu.
- Choose the case by clicking on *Case 4: 64-year-old-male—unknown medical.*
- Listen to the dispatch, or read it in the right panel (or both).
- Click **Start** and watch the entire video. Once the video has concluded, you are "on scene."

7. As the paramedics in this case begin their assessment of Jake, he asks them to just leave him alone. Should the paramedics leave him? Why or why not?

8. Assume that Jake is in the custody of law enforcement when the paramedics arrive. Jake asks them to just leave him alone. Should the paramedics leave him alone? Why or why not?

9. Jake awakens and becomes oriented after treatment. Jake refuses treatment after awakening. Should the paramedics permit Jake to refuse treatment? If the paramedics permit Jake to refuse treatment, what should be done?

10. Jake agrees to be transported to the hospital for an evaluation. When giving the report to the triage nurse, the paramedic characterizes Jake in an unfavorable way that results in Jake being sent to the waiting room to "wait his turn." What has the paramedic done?

• Click **Quit Case** and you will be taken to the summary menu.
• Click **Exit** to close the program, or **Restart** to continue with another lesson.

EXERCISE 3

 CD-ROM Activity

 Time: 15 minutes

 • Click **Restart** from the summary menu.
• Choose the case by clicking on *Case 9: 22-year-old-female—assault.*
• Listen to the dispatch, or read it in the right panel (or both).
• Click **Start** and watch the entire video. Once the video has concluded, you are "on scene."

11. As the paramedics in this case approach the patient, the police officer gives a summary of the patient's history of events leading up to the injury and review of injuries. Is the police officer's report sufficient? Why or why not?

12. As the paramedics begin their assessment, the patient indicates that she does not wish to be touched. What is further touching without permission called? Detail your plan for how you might handle this sudden change of heart by the patient.

13. Detail your course of action if law enforcement had not been at the location on arrival in this case.

- Click **Quit Case** and you will be taken to the summary menu.
- Click **Exit** to close the program, or **Restart** to continue with another lesson.

Ethics

👓 **Reading Assignment:** Read Chapter 5, Ethics, in *Paramedic Practice Today: Above and Beyond*.

Case 5: 40-year-old male—vomiting blood

Case 14: 65-year-old male—difficulty breathing

Objective:

On completion of this lesson, the student will be able to perform the following:

• Describe strategies to resolve ethical conflicts.

EXERCISE 1

 CD-ROM Activity

 Time: 15 minutes

- Sign into the software by entering your name in the name tag and clicking **Enter.**
- Choose the case by clicking on *Case 5: 40-year-old male—vomiting blood.*
- Listen to the dispatch, or read it in the right panel (or both).
- Click **Start** and watch the entire video. Once the video has concluded, you are "on scene."
- Read the history log on the right side of the screen.

1. Your patient is found behind a bar and complains of abdominal pain that began while he was drinking heavily. What moral or ethical dilemma might the paramedics have to overcome while treating this patient? How should the paramedics work through their dilemma?

2. During treatment, the patient in this case becomes uncooperative, insisting that the paramedics leave him to die. What are the ways in which the paramedics could deal with the patient's wishes?

3. On your return to the station, your colleagues want to know if the patient was intoxicated "again." What should your response be?

4. Law enforcement is investigating a report of an assault, and your patient is of interest to them. How should the interaction with law enforcement be handled?

5. You are contacted by the training officer and asked to review this case with some of your peers in an educational setting. How should you respond to this request?

 • Click **Quit Case** and you will be taken to the summary menu.
   • Click **Exit** to close the program, or **Restart** to continue with another lesson.

EXERCISE 2

 CD-ROM Activity

 Time: 15 minutes

 • Click **Restart** from the summary menu.
   • Choose the case by clicking on *Case 14: 65-year-old male—difficulty breathing.*
   • Listen to the dispatch, or read it in the right panel (or both).
   • Click **Start** and watch the entire video. Once the video has concluded, you are "on scene."
   • Read the history log on the right side of the screen.

6. What is your general impression of Patrick?

7. Patrick indicates to you he has a do not resuscitate order. You are unable to locate the document. What should your direction be? You are able to locate the DNR order, but it is unsigned. What should your direction be in this case?

8. What do you believe is in Patrick's best interest?

- Click **Quit Case** and you will be taken to the summary menu.
- Click **Exit** to close the program, or **Restart** to continue with another lesson.

LESSON 6

Medical Terminology Review

/OTD **Reading Assignment:** Read Chapter 6, Medical Terminology Review, in *Paramedic Practice Today: Above and Beyond.*.

Case 1: 20-year-old male—difficulty breathing

Case 2: 56-year-old female—fell

Case 10: 25-year-old female—abdominal pain

Case 14: 65-year-old male—difficulty breathing

Objectives:

On completion of this lesson, the student will be able to perform the following:

- Explain the importance of using correct medical terminology as it relates to each case.
- Demonstrate the ability to pronounce medical terms correctly.
- Describe the effect on patient care when a paramedic has a solid grasp of correct medical terminology.

31

EXERCISE 1

  CD-ROM Activity

 Time: 15 minutes

- Sign into the software by entering your name in the name tag and clicking **Enter.**
- Choose the case by clicking on *Case 1: 20-year-old male—difficulty breathing.*
- Listen to the dispatch, or read it in the right panel (or both).
- Click **Start** and watch the entire video. Once the video has concluded, you are "on scene."
- Read the history log on the right side of the screen.

1. James is suffering from a severe allergic reaction. What is the term for this reaction, and what does the word mean?

2. Does the name of the condition James is suffering from have a synonym? An antonym?

3. James has difficulty breathing as well. What word should the paramedic record when referring to James's difficultly breathing?

- Click **Quit Case,** and you will be taken to the summary menu.

EXERCISE 2

 CD-ROM Activity

 Time: 15 minutes

- Click **Restart** from the summary screen.
- Choose the case by clicking on *Case 2: 56-year-old female—fell.*
- Listen to the dispatch, or read it in the right panel (or both).
- Click **Start** and watch the entire video. Once the video has concluded, you are "on scene."
- Read the history log on the right side of the screen.

4. Describe how the patient is found in this case.

5. She woke up with labored breathing, which is often referred to as what? What is a common cause of this condition?

6. Her husband states his wife collapsed onto the floor, a condition known as *cardiac syncope.* What is cardiac syncope?

7. Using correct medical terminology, describe her appearance.

8. When the paramedic asks the husband about medications, he hands the paramedic a shoebox full of medications. Using your newfound knowledge about medical terminology, define *polypharmacy*.

 • Click **Quit Case,** and you will be taken to the summary menu.

EXERCISE 3

 CD-ROM Activity

 Time: 15 minutes

 • Click **Restart** from the summary screen.
• Choose the case by clicking on *Case 10: 25-year-old female—abdominal pain.*
• Listen to the dispatch, or read it in the right panel (or both).
• Click **Start** and watch the entire video. Once the video has concluded, you are "on scene."
• Read the history log on the right side of the screen.

9. The patient in this case has 1 month before she can be expected to deliver. Based on the nature of her complaint, her history of past pregnancies, and her prenatal care, prepare a short written report using correct medical terminology.

10. Based on the signs and symptoms available to you, what would your field impression of this patient be? What is the definition of the condition?

 • Click **Quit Case,** and you will be taken to the summary menu.

EXERCISE 4

 CD-ROM Activity

 Time: 15 minutes

 • Click **Restart** from the summary screen.
- Choose the case by clicking on *Case 14: 65-year-old male—difficulty breathing.*
- Listen to the dispatch, or read it in the right panel (or both).
- Click **Start** and watch the entire video. Once the video has concluded, you are "on scene."
- Read the history log on the right side of the screen.

11. Patrick is found sitting forward with his hands placed on his knees, and his work of breathing is increased. How would you describe your initial impression of Patrick?

12. What is increased work of breathing or difficult breathing commonly called?

13. The paramedics should be able to assume that Patrick is chronically ill based on his use of oxygen. What disease processes might be a cause of Patrick's difficult breathing? What is the disease?

Disease Name	Short Description

➤ • Click **Quit Case** and you will be taken to the summary menu.
   • Click **Exit** to close the program, or **Restart** to continue with another lesson.

Body Systems: Anatomy and Physiology

📖 **Reading Assignment:** Read Chapter 7, Body Systems: Anatomy and Physiology, in *Paramedic Practice Today: Above and Beyond.*

Case 11: 32-year-old male—gunshot wounds

Objectives:

On completion of this lesson, the student will be able to perform the following:

- Use directional terms appropriately to describe wound locations.
- Relate the observed injuries to the anatomic structures involved.
- Describe alterations in the physiologic condition that should be anticipated based on the wounds observed.

EXERCISE 1

CD-ROM Activity

Time: 10 minutes

→
- Sign into the software by entering your name in the name tag and clicking **Enter.**
- Choose the case by clicking on *Case 11: 32-year-old male—gunshot wounds.*
- Listen to the dispatch, or read it in the right panel (or both).
- Click **Start** and watch the entire video. Once the video has concluded, you are "on scene."
- Read the history log on the right side of the screen.

1. Describe the location of the injuries using proper anatomic terminology.

    a. The neck wound was located _____ to the midline of the neck.

    b. The chest wound was located _____ to the nipple and

    _____ to the clavicle.

    c. The abdominal wound was located _____ and

    _____ to the umbilicus. The abdominal wound was located in

    the _____ quadrant of the abdomen.

    d. The patient was found in the _____ position.

2. Predict which anatomic structures should be located under each wound:

    a. Neck wound:

    b. Chest wound:

c. Abdominal wound:

3. Predict alterations in the normal physiologic condition of body systems that may be affected by these wounds:

a. Neck wound:

b. Chest wound:

c. Abdominal wound:

 4. Using the dermatome map on page 152 of your textbook, predict the location where the patient would lose sensation if the neck wound penetrated the spinal cord.

→ • Click **Quit Case** and you will be taken to the summary menu.
  • Click **Exit** to close the program, or **Restart** to continue with another lesson.

Pathophysiology

✐ **Reading Assignment:** Read Chapter 8, Pathophysiology, in *Paramedic Practice Today: Above and Beyond.*

Case 1: 20-year-old male—difficulty breathing

Case 5: 40-year-old male—vomiting blood

Case 13: 5-month-old male—unresponsive

Objectives:

On completion of this lesson, the student will be able to perform the following:

- Predict alterations in pH that will be present based on the initial case information.
- Predict physiologic responses that will occur as the body compensates for acute blood volume loss.

EXERCISE 1

 CD-ROM Activity

 Time: 15 minutes

- Sign into the software by entering your name in the name tag and clicking **Enter.**
- Choose the case by clicking on *Case 1: 20-year-old male—difficulty breathing.*
- Listen to the dispatch, or read it in the right panel (or both).
- Click **Start** and watch the entire video. Once the video has concluded, you are "on scene."
- Read the history log on the right side of the screen.
- Click **Quit Case,** and you will be taken to the summary menu.
- Click **Restart**.
- Choose the next case by clicking on *Case 13: 5-month-old male—unresponsive.*
- Listen to the dispatch, watch the video, and read the history log for this case, too.

1. What alterations in blood gasses would you expect to find in each of these cases based on the initial information you are given for these calls?

Case	Partial Pressure of Oxygen (PO₂)		Partial Pressure of Carbon Dioxide (PCO₂)		pH	
	Alteration	Based on	Alteration	Based on	Alteration	Based on
1						
13						

2. What actions will you need to take to correct these alterations?

   a. Case 1:

   b. Case 13:

 • Click **Quit Case** and you will be taken to the summary menu.
   • Click **Exit** to close the program, or **Restart** to continue with another lesson.

EXERCISE 2

 CD-ROM Activity

 Time: 15 minutes

 • Click **Restart** on the summary menu.
   • Choose the case by clicking on *Case 5: 40-year-old male—vomiting blood.*
   • Listen to the dispatch, or read it in the right panel (or both).
   • Click **Start** and watch the entire video. Once the video has concluded, you are "on scene."
   • Read the history log on the right side of the screen.

3. Assume that, after assessing this patient, you determine he has the following vital signs: blood pressure (BP) 100/84, pulse (P) 128, respiration (R) 28, and skin is pale and cool. Is this compensated or uncompensated shock? Explain your answer.

4. Describe how the compensatory mechanisms activated in response to the patient's acute blood loss produce some of the physical findings of your examination.

Compensatory Mechanism	Action	Physical Finding
Increased sympathetic stimulation		
Adrenal medullary mechanism		
Aldosterone release		
Antidiuretic hormone (ADH)		

5. Which compensatory mechanisms increase intravascular volume during shock?

• Click **Quit Case** and you will be taken to the summary menu.
• Click **Exit** to close the program, or **Restart** to continue with another lesson.

Life Span Development

Reading Assignment: Read Chapter 9, Life Span Development, in *Paramedic Practice Today: Above and Beyond*.

Case 13: 5-month-old male—unresponsive

Case 6: 16-year-old female—unknown medical

Objectives:

On completion of this lesson, the student will be able to perform the following:

- Determine whether the children in these scenarios fall within normal age-specific developmental guidelines.
- Discuss the effect of emotional development on wellness.
- Distinguish between illnesses and injuries that occur within specific age ranges.

EXERCISE 1

 CD-ROM Activity

 Time: 20 minutes

- Sign into the software by entering your name in the name tag and clicking **Enter.**
- Choose the case by clicking on *Case 13: 5-month-old male—unresponsive.*
- Listen to the dispatch, or read it in the right panel (or both).
- Click **Start** and watch the entire video. Once the video has concluded, you are "on scene."
- Read the history log on the right side of the screen.

1. Does this infant's weight (16 lb) seem appropriate for a baby of his age? Explain your answer.

2. Would you have expected a 5-month-old infant to sleep through the night, or is the mother's story questionable?

3. If you resuscitate this baby, what vital signs would you expect as normal for his age?

4. If you resuscitate this baby and he becomes fully conscious, how would you expect him to respond to his mother?

5. How is a baby this age protected against disease?

6. If you resuscitate this child and stroke the outside of his foot and his toes fan up toward his head, how would you interpret these findings? What assessment have you performed?

7. Which of the following illnesses or injuries would you expect to find in a 5-month-old infant? If you said you would not expect it, then explain your answer.

Illness or Injury	Expected in a 5-Month-Old Infant	If You Said *No*, Explain Why
Father says infant burned his feet stepping into the tub		
Fell while walking and hit his head		
Choked on a bead		

 • Click **Quit Case,** and you will be taken to the summary menu.

EXERCISE 2

 CD-ROM Activity

 Time: 10 minutes

- Click **Restart** from the summary menu.
- Choose the case by clicking on *Case 6: 16-year-old female—unknown medical.*
- Listen to the dispatch, or read it in the right panel (or both).
- Click **Start** and watch the entire video. Once the video has concluded, you are "on scene."
- Read the history log on the right side of the screen.
- Assess one set of vital signs by clicking the appropriate **Assessment** buttons.

8. Do the patient's vital signs fall within the expected normal range for her age? Explain your answer.

9. What sexual characteristics should have developed in a girl of this age? Explain why this patient may have delayed development in this area.

10. What emotional developmental characteristics would predispose a girl of this age to develop anorexia?

11. What factors may lead you to believe that this situation is a suicide attempt?

  • Click **Quit Case,** and go to the summary menu.
    • Click **Exit** to close the program, or **Restart** to continue with another lesson.

Public Health and EMS

Reading Assignment: Read Chapter 10, Public Health and EMS, in *Paramedic Practice Today: Above and Beyond*.

Other Relevant Chapters:

- Chapter 7, Body Systems: Anatomy and Physiology
- Chapter 8, Pathophysiology

Case 15: 42-year-old male—difficulty breathing

Objectives:

On completion of this lesson, the student will be able to perform the following:

- Discuss the role of public health in preventing the spread of communicable disease.
- Describe the role of EMS in preventing the spread of communicable diseases.

EXERCISE 1

 CD-ROM Activity

 Time: 15 minutes

- Sign into the software by enter your name in the name tag and clicking **Enter.**
- Choose the case by clicking on *Case 15: 42-year-old male—difficulty breathing.*
- Listen to the dispatch, or read it in the right panel (or both).
- Click **Start** and watch the entire video. Once the video has concluded, you are "on scene."
- Read the history log on the right of the screen.

1. What types of masks should the crew use when treating this patient?

2. Upon arrival at the hospital, what should the crew do to minimize the risk to hospital staff members and patients?

3. What should the paramedics do if the patient is noncompliant with medications or is not under the care of a physician?

- Click **Quit Case,** and go to the summary menu.
- Click **Exit** to close the program, or **Restart** to continue with another lesson.

Basic Principles of Pharmacology

Reading Assignment: Read Chapter 11, Basic Principles of Pharmacology, in *Paramedic Practice Today: Above and Beyond.*

Case 1: 20-year-old male—difficulty breathing

Objectives:

On completion of this lesson, the student will be able to perform the following:

- Recognize the role of medication identification in determining the clinical impression.
- Describe the role of receptors and how medications interact with receptors to generate physiologic responses.
- Value the importance of interpreting patient medication therapy as part of the assessment process.

EXERCISE 1

 CD-ROM Activity

 Time: 15 minutes

- Sign in at the software by entering your name in the name tag and clicking **Enter.**
- Choose the case by clicking on *Case 1: 20-year-old male—difficulty breathing.*
- Listen to the dispatch, or read it in the right panel (or both).
- Click **Start** and watch the entire video. Once the video has concluded, you are "on scene."
- Read the history log on the right side of the screen.

1. What is the clinical significance of the patient having an EpiPen?

2. With what receptors does the drug epinephrine interact, and what are the effects of those interactions?

Receptor	Effect	Clinical Evidence

- Click **Quit Case,** and go to the summary menu.
- Click **Exit** to close the program, or **Restart** to continue with another lesson.

Drug and Chemical Classes

✐ **Reading Assignment:** Read Chapter 12, Drug and Chemical Classes, in *Paramedic Practice Today: Above and Beyond.*

Other Relevant Chapters:

• Chapter 11, Basic Principles of Pharmacology

Case 2: 56-year-old female—fell

Case 4: 64-year-old male—unknown medical

Case 12: 57-year-old male—man down

Case 5: 40-year-old male—vomiting blood

Objectives:

On completion of this lesson, the student will be able to perform the following:

• Recognize the role of medication identification in determining the clinical impression.

• Distinguish onset, peak, and duration of action of various types of insulin.

• Outline the actions of various types of antihypertensive medications.

• Value the importance of interpreting patient medication therapy as part of the assessment process.

• Be familiar with the profiles of commonly prescribed medications.

EXERCISE 1

 CD-ROM Activity

 Time: 15 minutes

- Sign into the software by entering your name in the name tag and clicking **Enter.**
- Choose the case by clicking on *Case 2: 56-year-old female—fell.*
- Listen to the dispatch, or read it in the right panel (or both).
- Click **Start** and watch the entire video. Once the video has concluded, you are "on scene."
- Read the history log on the right side of the screen.

1. What historical information missing on the call could have assisted you in making a clinical decision?

2. Assuming that this patient's husband gave the paramedic the medications listed in each of the following examples, find each of the drugs in Appendix B, Drug Profiles, at the back of your textbook, in the "Drug Guide" in the software, or in Mosby's Essential Drug List for *Paramedic Practice Today* on Evolve (http://evolve.elsevier.com/Aehlert/paramedic). Then identify the class of the drug and what conditions each drug is used to treat. Finally, under "Impression," list some possible causes of the patient's difficulty breathing, based on this information.

EXAMPLE 1 (same medications as listed in the history in the software)

Medications	Drug Class	Medicines Prescribed for
Lanoxin		
Bumex		
Hydrochlorothiazide		
Serevent		
Albuterol		
Impression:		

EXAMPLE 2

Medications	Drug Class	Medicines Prescribed for
Coreg		
Spironolactone		
Diovan		
Furosemide		
Impression:		

EXAMPLE 3

Medications	Drug Class	Medicines Prescribed for
Rifampin		
Isoniazid		
Combivent		
Impression:		

EXAMPLE 4

Medications	Drug Class	Medicines Prescribed for
Singulair		
Maxair		
Advair		
Impression:		

EXAMPLE 5

Medications	Drug Class	Medicines Prescribed for
Isosorbide		
Persantine		
Lipitor		
Accupril		
Impression:		

EXAMPLE 6

Medications	Drug Class	Medicines Prescribed for
Combivir		
Indinavir (Crixivan)		
Impression:		

EXAMPLE 7

Medications	Drug Class	Medicines Prescribed for
Metformin		
Avalide		
Repaglinide (Prandin)		
Impression:		

➤ • Click **Quit Case,** and you will be taken to the summary menu.

EXERCISE 2

 CD-ROM Activity

 Time: 15 minutes

- Click **Restart** from the summary menu.
- Choose the case by clicking on *Case 4: 64-year-old male—unknown medical.*
- Listen to the dispatch, or read it in the right panel (or both).
- Click **Start** and watch the entire video. Once the video has concluded, you are "on scene."
- Read the history log on the right side of the screen.

3. You find a medication list on this patient's refrigerator that indicates he is taking insulin. Fill in the missing information related to the generic or trade name, and then list how long it takes to achieve the peak effect and the duration of the effect of each of the following insulins when administered subcutaneously.

Generic Name	Trade Name	Onset of Effect	Peak Effect	Duration
	Humulin U			
Insulin recombinant human				
	Lantus			
Insulin aspart recombinant				
	Apidra			

4. Which of the insulins listed in the previous table may be given by insulin pump?

5. Why is it important to know the time of onset, peak action, and duration for each insulin?

 • Click **Quit Case,** and you will be taken to the summary menu.

EXERCISE 3

 CD-ROM Activity

 Time: 15 minutes

 • Click **Restart** from the summary menu.
• Choose the case by clicking on *Case 12: 57-year-old male—man down.*
• Listen to the dispatch, or read it in the right panel (or both).
• Click **Start** and watch the entire video. Once the video has concluded, you are "on scene."
• Read the history log on the right side of the screen.

6. The patient in this case is taking two antihypertensive agents, Vasotec and Bumex. Many types of drugs are used to treat hypertension. Complete the information in the following table related to these and other antihypertensive agents.

Generic Name	Trade Name	Drug Classification	Action
Doxazosin			
	Vasotec		

Generic Name	Trade Name	Drug Classification	Action
Irbesartan			
	Toprol XL		
Amlodipine			
	Bumex		
	Hydrodiuril		

→ • Click **Quit Case,** and you will be taken to the summary menu.

EXERCISE 4

 CD-ROM Activity

 Time: 15 minutes

→ • Click **Restart** from the summary menu.
• Choose the case by clicking on *Case 5: 40-year-old male—vomiting blood.*
• Listen to the dispatch, or read it in the right panel (or both).
• Click **Start** and watch the entire video. Once the video has concluded, you are "on scene."
• Read the history log on the right side of the screen.

[]

7. Describe how this patient's present illness and medical history will affect drug absorption, distribution, and biotransformation, as well as how these could affect drug therapy if it were indicated.

	Absorption	Distribution	Biotransformation
Illness effects on each			
Impact on drug treatment (if indicated)			

 • Click **Quit Case,** and you will be taken to the summary menu.

EXERCISE 5

 CD-ROM Activity

 Time: 10 minutes

 • Sign into the software by entering your name in the name tag and clicking **Enter.**
• Choose the case by clicking on *Case 6: 16-year-old male—unknown medical.*
• Listen to the dispatch, or read it in the right panel (or both).
• Click **Start** and watch the entire video. Once the video has concluded, you are "on scene."
• Read the history log on the right side of the screen.

8. What elements of patient history are clinically important in this case?

 • Click **Exit** to close the program, or **Restart** to continue with another lesson.

Medication Administration

Reading Assignment: Read Chapter 13, Medication Administration, in *Paramedic Practice Today: Above and Beyond.*

Case 5: 40-year-old male—vomiting blood

Case 13: 5-month-old male—unresponsive

Case 12: 57-year-old male—man down

Objectives:

On completion of this lesson, the student will be able to perform the following:

- Determine appropriate situations for the use of intraosseous infusion.
- Identify appropriate medication administration routes based on an understanding of life span development.
- Calculate drug doses accurately.

EXERCISE 1

 CD-ROM Activity

 Time: 10 minutes

- Sign into the software by entering your name in the name tag and clicking **Enter.**
- Choose the case by clicking on *Case 5: 40-year-old male—vomiting blood.*
- Listen to the dispatch, or read it in the right panel (or both).
- Click **Start** and watch the entire video. Once the video has concluded, you are "on scene."
- Read the history log on the right side of the screen.
- Click **Quit Case,** and you will be taken to the summary menu.
- Click **Restart** and choose another case by clicking on *Case 13: 5-month-old male— unresponsive.*
- Listen to the dispatch, or read it in the right panel (or both).
- Click **Start** and watch the entire video. Once the video has concluded, you are "on scene."
- Read the history log on the right side of the screen.

For the first four questions, assume you are unable to establish intravenous (IV) access in both of these cases and answer the following questions.

1. Would the intraosseous route be an acceptable vascular access route in each of these cases?

   a. Case 5:

   b. Case 13:

2. At what point would you elect to perform intraosseous access in each of these cases?

   a. Case 5:

   b. Case 13:

3. Why is the intraosseous route preferred over the endotracheal route?

   a. Case 5:

   b. Case 13:

4. In each of the two cases (assuming the patient has a pulse and is perfusing well), describe an appropriate site for administration of an intramuscular injection.

   a. Case 5:

   b. Case 13:

   For the next three questions, assume that the patient in each case needs the following interventions and that the adult weights 220 lb and the child weighs 15 lb.

5. Assume that you want to administer dopamine 5 mcg/kg/min. You have 200 mg dopamine in 250 mL D_5W. Your IV tubing drop factor is 60 gtt/mL. How many drops per minute will you run your fluid?

   a. Case 5:

   b. Case 13:

6. Assume you want to administer lidocaine 2 mg/min to the patient in Case 5. You have 1 g lidocaine in 250 mL D₅W. Your IV tubing drop factor is 60 gtt/mL. How many drops per minute will you run your fluid?

7. Assume you want to administer 20 mL/kg fluid bolus over 20 minutes to the patient in Case 13. Your IV tubing drop factor is 20 gtt/mL. How many drops per minute will you run your fluid?

 • Click **Quit Case,** and you will be taken to the summary menu.

EXERCISE 2

 CD-ROM Activity

 Time: 15 minutes

 • Click **Restart** from the summary menu.
• Choose the case by clicking on *Case 12: 57-year-old male—man down.*
• Listen to the dispatch, or read it in the right panel (or both).
• Click **Start** and watch the entire video. Once the video has concluded, you are "on scene."
• Read the history log on the right side of the screen.

8. Assume that you determined the patient needed the following drugs and dosing schedule after you completed your history and physical examination and determined your diagnosis. Identify the proper route of administration, then calculate the correct volume or drip rate to administer. Assume that the macrodrip IV tubing delivers 10 gtt/mL.

Condition	Drug and Dose	Route	Volume (or gtt/min) to Administer
Dehydration	Normal saline 250 mL over 20 min		

Condition	Drug and Dose	Route	Volume (or gtt/min) to Administer
Hypoglycemia	25 g 50% Dextrose		
OxyContin overdose	Naloxone 0.8 mg IV (supplied as 2 mg in 2 mL)		
Nausea and vomiting	Promethazine 12.5 mg (supplied as 50 mg/mL)		

 • Click **Quit Case,** and you will be taken to the summary menu.
• Click **Exit** to close the program, or **Restart** to continue with another lesson.

LESSON 14

Airway Management

Reading Assignment: Read Chapter 14, Airway Management, in *Paramedic Practice Today: Above and Beyond*.

Case 1: 20-year-old male—difficulty breathing

Case 2: 56-year-old female—fell

Case 5: 40-year-old male—vomiting blood

Case 6: 16-year-old female—unknown medical

Objectives:

On completion of this lesson, the student will be able to perform the following:

- Assess and manage an airway obstruction.
- Use preventive measures for pulmonary aspiration.
- Evaluate the airway for patency and breathing for adequacy.

71

Copyright © 2010 by Mosby, Inc., an affiliate of Elsevier Inc. All rights reserved.

EXERCISE 1

Preparation Activity

Time: 10 minutes

- Before beginning the simulation, review the Fick principle on page 233 of your textbook.

1. What conditions or diseases might reduce the oxygen available for exchange at the alveolar level?

2. List ways in which a patient might be treated for low oxygen levels.

3. What conditions or diseases impair circulation of red blood cells to the tissue?

4. List ways in which a patient might be treated for impaired circulation.

5. What conditions or diseases impair the exchange of oxygen and carbon dioxide at the alveolar level and again at the cellular level?

6. List ways in which a patient might be treated for impaired oxygen–carbon dioxide exchange.

EXERCISE 2

 CD-ROM Activity

 Time: 20 minutes

→
- Sign into the software by entering your name in the name tag and clicking **Enter.**
- Choose the case by clicking on *Case 1: 20-year-old male—difficulty breathing.*
- Listen to the dispatch, or read it in the right panel (or both).
- Click **Start** and watch the entire video. Once the video has concluded, you are "on scene."
- Read the history log on the right side of the screen.
- Perform your initial assessment using the **Assessment** buttons in the left panel.

7. What is causing James's difficulty breathing?

8. What would the benefit be for James if oxygen were applied?

9. Did pulse oximetry provide useful information in this case? Why or why not?

10. Would capnography provide useful information in this case? Why or why not?

- Click **Quit Case,** and you will be taken to the summary menu.
- Click on **Log**.
- To save your log, click on the disk icon. To print your log, click on the printer icon.
- Click **Menu** to return to the summary menu.

EXERCISE 3

 CD-ROM Activity

 Time: 20 minutes

→ • Click **Restart** from the summary menu.
   • Choose the case by clicking on *Case 2: 56-year-old female—fell.*
   • Listen to the dispatch, or read it in the right panel (or both).
   • Click **Start** and watch the entire video. Once the video has concluded, you are "on scene."
   • Read the history log on the right side of the screen.
   • Perform your initial assessment using the **Assessment** buttons in the left panel.

11. List the signs of respiratory distress that you observe in this patient.

12. The original dispatch was for a woman who fell. List possible causes of her dyspnea.

13. List physiologic concerns that might make management of this patient's airway, oxygenation, and ventilation more difficult.

14. Did pulse oximetry provide valuable information in this patient? Why or why not?

15. Would capnography provide valuable information in this patient? Why or why not?

 • Click **Quit Case,** and you will be taken to the summary menu.
• Click on **Log**.
• To save your log, click on the disk icon. To print your log, click on the printer icon.
• Click **Menu** to return to the summary menu.

EXERCISE 4

 CD-ROM Activity

 Time: 20 minutes

 • Click **Restart** from the summary menu.
• Choose the case by clicking on *Case 5: 40-year-old male—vomiting blood.*
• Listen to the dispatch, or read it in the right panel (or both).

 16. Before beginning the video, review the steps for suctioning, Skills 14-1 and 14-2 of your textbook, and list below.

 • Click **Start** and watch the entire video. Once the video has concluded, you are "on scene."
• Read the history log on the right side of the screen.
• Perform your initial assessment using the **Assessment** buttons in the left panel.

17. What concerns do you have about this patient's airway?

18. How would you prepare yourself to care for this patient's airway?

19. Did pulse oximetry provide useful information in this case? Why or why not?

20. Would capnography provide useful information in this case? Why or why not?

 • Click **Quit Case,** and you will be taken to the summary menu.
• Click on **Log**.
• To save your log, click on the disk icon. To print your log, click on the printer icon.
• Click **Menu** to return to the summary menu.

EXERCISE 5

 CD-ROM Activity

 Time: 20 minutes

 • Click **Restart** from the summary menu.
• Choose the case by clicking on *Case 6: 16-year-old female—unknown medical.*
• Listen to the dispatch, or read it in the right panel (or both).

 21. Before beginning the video, review the steps for insertion of the nasopharyngeal airway in Skill 14-4 of your textbook and list below.

• Click **Start** and watch the entire video. Once the video has concluded, you are "on scene."
 • Read the history log on the right side of the screen.
 • Perform your initial assessment using the **Assessment** buttons in the left panel.

22. What are your management priorities for Sarah?

23. Would pulse oximetry provide valuable information on Sarah? Why or why not?

24. Would capnography provide valuable information on Sarah? Why or why not?

 • Click **Quit Case,** and you will be taken to the summary menu.
 • Click on **Log**.
 • To save your log, click on the disk icon. To print your log, click on the printer icon.
 • Click **Menu** to return to the summary menu.
 • Click **Exit** to close the program, or **Restart** to continue with another lesson

15 _____

Therapeutic Communication

_____

/OTO **Reading Assignment:** Read Chapter 15, Therapeutic Communication, in *Paramedic Practice Today: Above and Beyond.*

Case 2: 56-year-old female—fell

Case 9: 22-year-old female—assault

Case 10: 25-year-old female—abdominal pain

Objectives:

On completion of this lesson, the student will be able to perform the following:

- Identify therapeutic communication techniques used by the paramedics in selected cases.
- Recognize barriers to effective communication and identify strategies that may be used to overcome them.

EXERCISE 1

 CD-ROM Activity

 Time: 15 minutes

- Sign into the software by entering your name in the name tag and clicking **Enter.**
- Choose the case by clicking on *Case 2: 56-year-old female—fell.*
- Listen to the dispatch, or read it in the right panel (or both).
- Click **Start** and watch the entire video. Once the video has concluded, you are "on scene."
- Read the history log on the right side of the screen.

1. Review the steps for effective communication involved in the LADDER of listening. Describe whether you observed each step in this case.

	Techniques for Effective Listening	How the Techniques Are Demonstrated
L		
A		
D		
D		
E		
R		

2. What barrier to effective therapeutic communication existed in this case?

3. How can paramedics adapt to this barrier most effectively?

 • Click **Quit Case,** and you will be taken to the summary menu.

EXERCISE 2

 CD-ROM Activity

 Time: 15 minutes

 • Click **Restart** from the summary menu.
• Choose the case by clicking on *Case 9: 22-year-old female—assault.*
• Listen to the dispatch, or read it in the right panel (or both).
• Click **Start** and watch the entire video. Once the video has concluded, you are "on scene."
• Read the history log on the right side of the screen.

4. Describe the paramedic's communication with this patient as it relates to the following:

  a. Listening:

  b. Patience:

c. Providing privacy:

d. Eye contact:

e. Personal dress:

f. Touch:

5. What barriers to effective therapeutic communication existed on this call?

6. What strategies can paramedics use to overcome these barriers?

7. If the police officer had not been present, how might the officer's absence have affected the interview?

 • Click **Quit Case,** and you will be taken to the summary menu.

EXERCISE 3

 CD-ROM Activity

 Time: 15 minutes

 • Click **Restart** from the summary menu.
• Choose the case by clicking on *Case 10: 25-year-old female—abdominal pain.*
• Listen to the dispatch, or read it in the right panel (or both).
• Click **Start** and watch the entire video. Once the video has concluded, you are "on scene."
• Read the history log on the right side of the screen.

8. What barrier to communication was present on this case?

 9. Explain the techniques described on pages 572 to 573 of the textbook that the paramedic used with the interpreter to obtain the appropriate information.

10. If the interpreter had not been present, could the interpreter's absence have changed your clinical impression? Explain your answer.

11. What techniques could have been used to obtain information in the absence of an interpreter?

- Click **Quit Case,** and you will be taken to the summary menu.
- Click **Exit** to close the program, or **Restart** to continue with another lesson.

LESSON 16

History Taking

Reading Assignment: Read Chapter 16, History Taking, in *Paramedic Practice Today: Above and Beyond*.

Case 6: 16-year-old female—unknown medical
Case 14: 65-year-old male—difficulty breathing

Objectives:

On completion of this lesson, the student will be able to perform the following:

- Evaluate a patient within the context of additional information about the patient's history.
- Value the importance of patient history as part of the assessment process.

85

EXERCISE 1

 CD-ROM Activity

 Time: 15 minutes

- Sign into the software by entering your name in the name tag and clicking **Enter.**
- Choose the case by clicking on *Case 6: 16-year-old female—unknown medical.*
- Listen to the dispatch, or read it in the right panel (or both).
- Click **Start** and watch the entire video. Once the video has concluded, you are "on scene."
- Read the history log on the right side of the screen.

1. What physical findings would you anticipate if, after examining the pill bottle or after talking with the patient's parents, you discover the following information? What clinical impression or impressions would you consider as significant?

Information	Impressions	Physical Findings
Patient has been using oxycodone (OxyContin) and was released from drug rehabilitation last week.		
Her parents just discovered she is bulimic. Her weight is 60 lb. Her physician called when he received her laboratory results and told her parents to call an ambulance; he said that he would arrange for a direct admission to the intensive care unit (ICU).		
The patient wrote a suicide note; the bottle was filled with digoxin yesterday.		

Information	Impression	Physical Findings
Her parents tell you she is diabetic and has been vomiting for 2 days.		

 • Click **Quit Case,** and you will be taken to the summary menu.

EXERCISE 2

 CD-ROM Activity

 Time: 10 minutes

 • Click **Restart** from the summary menu.
- Choose the case by clicking on *Case 14: 65-year-old male—difficulty breathing.*
- Listen to the dispatch, or read it in the right panel (or both).
- Click **Start** and watch the entire video. Once the video has concluded, you are "on scene."
- Read the history log on the right side of the screen.

2. What form of questioning did the paramedic use to begin the interview of the patient?

3. After discovering the patient was having difficulty communicating, how did the paramedic change his questioning?

4. What nonverbal communication techniques did you notice during the initial assessment?

5. What physical findings would you anticipate if you discover the following information? What clinical impression or impressions would you consider as significant?

Information	Impressions	Physical Findings
Patient is drowsy, vomiting, and dyspneic, and he has a headache. His furnace has not been working correctly.		
He has noticed a cough with green sputum for several days. He is now febrile.		
The patient has a history of severe emphysema, and he has developed sudden dyspnea with a sharp pain in the right side of his chest.		
The patient's home medicines include an Atrovent inhaler, Singulair, a Maxair inhaler, and prednisone that he says his physician prescribed 2 days earlier.		

- Click **Quit Case,** and you will be taken to the summary menu.
- Click **Exit** to close the program, or **Restart** to continue with another lesson.

Patient Assessment I

Reading Assignment: Read Chapter 17, Patient Assessment, in *Paramedic Practice Today: Above and Beyond.*

Case 1: 20-year-old male—difficulty breathing
Case 2: 56-year-old female—fell
Case 3: 7-year-old female—seizure
Case 4: 64-year-old male—unknown medical
Case 5: 40-year-old male—vomiting blood
Case 6: 16-year-old female—unknown medical
Case 9: 22-year-old female—assault
Case 12: 57-year-old male—man down

Objectives:

On completion of this lesson, the student will be able to perform the following:

- Recall the components of patient assessment.
- Identify the essential patient assessment information from the scenario.
- Determine appropriate additional assessment needed.
- Discuss how to apply the phases of the patient assessment to each patient situation.

EXERCISE 1

Preparation Activity

Time: 15 minutes

Before you start the simulation, consider the priorities in the assessment information needed.

1. List the assessment priorities and information needed in the initial assessment.

2. List the assessment priorities and information needed in the focused assessment.

3. List the assessment priorities and information needed in the detailed assessment.

EXERCISE 2

CD-ROM Activity

Time: 15 minutes

- Sign into the software by entering your name in the name tag and clicking **Enter.**
- Choose the case by clicking on *Case 1: 20-year-old male—difficulty breathing.*
- Listen to the dispatch, or read it in the right panel (or both).
- Click **Start** and watch the entire video. Once the video has concluded, you are "on scene."
- Read the history log on the right side of the screen.

4. Why was it important to listen to the information provided by the emergency medical responders and by the resident advisor for the dormitory?

5. Using only the information you have from the initial dispatch and video information, identify the following:

   a. Your general impression of this patient:

   b. Patient's level of consciousness:

   c. Patient's airway status:

   d. Patient's oxygenation and respiratory status:

   e. Patient's circulatory status:

6. Predict the life threats (if any) you will need to treat during the initial assessment of this patient. Explain your rationale.

7. List at least three possible causes of the symptoms presented in this case.

→ • Click **Quit Case,** and you will be taken to the summary menu.

EXERCISE 3

 CD-ROM Activity

 Time: 15 minutes

 • Click **Restart** from the summary menu.
  • Choose the case by clicking on *Case 2: 56-year-old female—fell.*
  • Listen to the dispatch, or read it in the right panel (or both).
  • Click **Start** and watch the entire video. Once the video has concluded, you are "on scene."

8. What is your general impression of this patient?

9. What difficulties did the team encounter in obtaining the initial patient information?

10. How can the team overcome some of these difficulties?

 • Read the history log on the right side of the screen.

11. What additional assessment information will be needed for this patient?

12. List at least three possible causes of the signs and symptoms you have gathered up to this point for this case.

 • Click **Quit Case,** and you will be taken to the summary menu.

EXERCISE 4

 CD-ROM Activity

Time: 15 minutes

 • Click **Restart** from the summary menu.
• Choose the case by clicking on *Case 3: 7-year-old female—seizure.*
• Listen to the dispatch, or read it in the right panel (or both).
• Click **Start** and watch the entire video. Once the video has concluded, you are "on scene."
• Read the history log on the right side of the screen.

13. Describe the components of the scene size-up that you assessed on this case.

Component	Assessment
Nature	
Number of patients	
Hazards identified	
Additional resources needed	
Are access or staging areas identified?	
Is the area secure?	

14. During the video, the emergency medical services (EMS) team has gathered important assessment information. What is your general impression of this patient?

15. Do you have enough information to determine if this case is related to illness or trauma? Explain your answer.

 • Click **Quit Case,** and you will be taken to the summary menu.

EXERCISE 5

 CD-ROM Activity

 Time: 15 minutes

 • Click **Restart** from the summary menu.
• Choose the case by clicking on *Case 4: 64-year-old male—unknown medical.*
• Listen to the dispatch, or read it in the right panel (or both).
• Click **Start** and watch the entire video. Once the video has concluded, you are "on scene."

16. What information did the EMS team obtain during the scene size-up?

Component	Assessment
Nature	
Number of patients	
Hazards identified	
Additional resources needed	

Component	Assessment
Are access or staging areas identified?	
Is the area secure?	

17. What additional assessment information should you obtain on this patient?

 • Read the history log on the right side of the screen.

18. Based on the history log and your observations from the video, list at least four current differential diagnoses for this case.

 • Click **Quit Case,** and you will be taken to the summary menu.

EXERCISE 6

 CD-ROM Activity

 Time: 15 minutes

 • Click **Restart** from the summary menu.
  • Choose the case by clicking on *Case 5: 40-year-old male—vomiting blood.*
  • Listen to the dispatch, or read it in the right panel (or both).
  • Click **Start** and watch the entire video. Once the video has concluded, you are "on scene."
  • Read the history log on the right side of the screen.

19. Describe your scene size-up and assessment for this call.

Component	Assessment
Nature	
Number of patients	
Hazards identified	
Additional resources needed	
Are access or staging areas identified?	
Is the area secure?	

20. What personal protective equipment (PPE) is appropriate for this type of call?

21. What life threats do you anticipate you will find in your initial assessment of this patient, based on the information from the scene size-up?

22. Based on the information you have, will this person be a priority patient? Explain your answer.

23. What type of focused assessment will you perform on this patient?

24. What type of detailed physical examination would be performed on this patient?

25. What are the components of the ongoing assessment?

26. How often will you perform an ongoing assessment on this patient?

➡ • Click **Quit Case,** and you will be taken to the summary menu.

EXERCISE 7

 CD-ROM Activity

 Time: 15 minutes

- Click **Restart** from the summary menu.
- Choose the case by clicking on *Case 6: 16-year-old female—unknown medical.*
- Listen to the dispatch, or read it in the right panel (or both).
- Click **Start** and watch the entire video. Once the video has concluded, you are "on scene."
- Read the history log on the right side of the screen.

27. What interventions should you anticipate having to perform during the initial assessment, based on the information you presently have?

28. What additional information will you need to determine whether this is a priority patient?

29. List life threats that you would have anticipated if, instead of Elavil, the empty pill bottle had contained the following drugs.

Drug	Life Threats Anticipated
Heroin	
Digoxin	
Xanax	

Drug	Life Threats Anticipated
Metoprolol	
Verapamil	

 • Click **Quit Case,** and you will be taken to the summary menu.

EXERCISE 8

 CD-ROM Activity

 Time: 15 minutes

 • Click **Restart** from the summary menu.
- Choose the case by clicking on *Case 9: 22-year-old female—assault.*
- Listen to the dispatch, or read it in the right panel (or both).
- Click **Start** and watch the entire video. Once the video has concluded, you are "on scene."
- Read the history log on the right side of the screen.

During the video, the EMS team has gathered important assessment information that can be used to determine the nature of the situation. Based on the initial information from the police officers and from the patient, consider the following questions.

30. Did you note or do you expect to find any life threats related to level of consciousness, airway and breathing, and circulation?

31. What additional focused assessments should be performed on this patient?

32. What factors will interfere with your ability to perform a complete assessment of this patient?

 • Click **Quit Case,** and you will be taken to the summary menu.

EXERCISE 9

 CD-ROM Activity

 Time: 15 minutes

 • Click **Restart** from the summary menu.
• Choose the case by clicking on *Case 12: 57-year-old male—man down.*
• Listen to the dispatch, or read it in the right panel (or both).
• Click **Start** and watch the entire video. Once the video has concluded, you are "on scene."
• Read the history log on the right side of the screen.

33. What sources of information relative to the situation and the patient's condition did you have on this call?

34. What additional assessments should you perform on this patient?

35. What preliminary information do you have about his airway, breathing, and respiration status?

36. Explain whether capillary refill would or would not be a reliable assessment to perform on this patient.

37. List at least four possible causes of the signs and symptoms presented in this case.

• Click **Quit Case,** and you will be taken to the summary menu.
• Click **Exit** to close the program, or **Restart** to continue with another lesson.

Patient Assessment II

👓 **Reading Assignment:** Read Chapter 17, Patient Assessment, in *Paramedic Practice Today: Above and Beyond*.

Case 1: 20-year-old male—difficulty breathing

Case 2: 56-year-old female—fell

Case 10: 25-year-old female—abdominal pain

Objectives:

On completion of this lesson, the student will be able to perform the following:

- Demonstrate physical examination techniques in the given scenario.
- Describe the components of a comprehensive physical examination for the given scenario.
- Describe the general approach to a physical examination.
- Distinguish between normal and abnormal findings in a mental status assessment.
- Demonstrate physical examination techniques used for specific body regions.

EXERCISE 1

 Preparation Activity

Time: 10 minutes

1. Before you begin the simulation, recall the techniques of physical examination you will need to use. List and describe them here:

   a.

   b.

   c.

   d.

EXERCISE 2

 CD-ROM Activity

 Time: 15 minutes

- Sign into the software by entering your name in the name tag and clicking **Enter.**
- Choose the case by clicking on *Case 1: 20-year-old male—difficulty breathing.*
- Listen to the dispatch, or read it in the right panel (or both).
- Click **Start** and begin watching the video.
- Click **Pause (II)** as soon as the paramedic begins to listen to the patient's lung sounds.

2. What signs or symptoms should you anticipate with this type of complaint?

3. Describe a thorough assessment of James's chest.

→ • Click **Play** (▶), and let the video conclude—you are now "on scene."
  • Read the history log on the right side of the screen.

4. Why would you focus your physical assessment more on James's respiratory effort and thorax than on the rest of his body?

5. Describe your technique to auscultate James's thorax.

6. What sounds would you expect to hear as you auscultate James's thorax?

→ • Click **Quit Case,** and you will be taken to the summary menu.

EXERCISE 3

  CD-ROM Activity

 Time: 10 minutes

- Click **Restart** from the summary menu.
- Choose the case by clicking on *Case 2: 56-year-old female—fell.*
- Listen to the dispatch, or read it in the right panel (or both).
- Click **Start** and watch the entire video. Once the video has concluded, you are "on scene."

7. What signs of distress do you see in this patient?

8. How would you describe her initial mental status examination?

9. What are your immediate assessment priorities for this patient?

10. Which techniques of physical examination may need to be modified, based on your initial impression of this patient?

- Read the history log on the right side of the screen.
- Perform your initial assessment by clicking the appropriate **Assessment** buttons.

11. Based on your assessment of the patient, what type of illness or complaint do you suspect?

 • Click **Quit Case,** and you will be taken to the summary menu.

EXERCISE 4

 CD-ROM Activity

 Time: 10 minutes

 • Click **Restart** from the summary menu.
• Choose the case by clicking on *Case 10: 25-year-old female—abdominal pain.*
• Listen to the dispatch, or read it in the right panel (or both).
• Click **Start** and watch the entire video. Once the video has concluded, you are "on scene."

12. Describe the order in which you will perform examination techniques on the abdomen.

13. How will Connie's pregnancy affect your assessment of her abdomen?

 • Click **Quit Case,** and you will be taken to the summary menu.
• Click **Exit** to close the program, or **Restart** to continue with another lesson.

Communication

Reading Assignment: Read Chapter 18, Communication, in *Paramedic Practice Today: Above and Beyond*.

Case 2: 56-year-old female—fell

Case 7: 8-year-old male—submersion

Case 11: 32-year-old male—gunshot wounds

Objectives:

On completion of this lesson, the student will be able to perform the following:

- Explain the importance of the dispatch information.
- Describe the effects of inadequate or inappropriate dispatch information.

EXERCISE 1

 CD-ROM Activity

 Time: 15 minutes

→
- Sign into the software by entering your name in the name tag and clicking **Enter.**
- Choose the case by clicking on *Case 2: 56-year-old female—fell.*
- Listen to the dispatch, or read it in the right panel (or both).
- Click **Start** and watch the entire video. Once the video has concluded, you are "on scene."
- Read the history log on the right side of the screen.

1. Did the dispatch complaint relate directly to the patient's chief complaint?

2. Why might the dispatch information be inaccurate?

3. Could the dispatch information affect what equipment these paramedics bring into the patient's home? Explain your answer.

4. Did the paramedics focus on the dispatch information as the chief cause of illness? Explain your answer.

5. How could incorrect dispatch information delay the response to the scene?

6. After the paramedic spoke with the patient's husband, what information should he have communicated to his partner?

 • Click **Quit Case,** and you will be taken to the summary menu.

EXERCISE 2

 CD-ROM Activity

 Time: 10 minutes

 • Click **Restart** from the summary menu.
• Choose the case by clicking on *Case 7: 8-year-old male—submersion.*
• Listen to the dispatch, or read it in the right panel (or both).
• Click **Start** and watch the entire video. Once the video has concluded, you are "on scene."
• Read the history log on the right side of the screen.
• Click **Quit Case,** and you will be taken to the summary menu.
• Click **Restart** from the summary menu.
• Repeat the previous steps for *Case 11: 32-year-old male—gunshot wounds.*

7. What effect could incorrect dispatch information have had in each of these cases?

   a. Case 7:

b. Case 11:

8. If the dispatch information sounds odd to you, then what should you do in each of these cases?

a. Case 7:

b. Case 11:

➡ • Click **Quit Case,** and go to the summary menu.
• Click **Exit** to close the program, or **Restart** to continue with another lesson.

Documentation

Reading Assignment: Read Chapter 19, Documentation, in *Paramedic Practice Today: Above and Beyond.*

Case 1: 20-year-old male—difficulty breathing

Case 11: 32-year-old male—gunshot wounds

Case 9: 22-year-old female—assault

Case 14: 65-year-old male—difficulty breathing

Case 13: 5-month-old male—unresponsive

Case 8: 38-year-old male—suicide attempt

Objectives:

On completion of this lesson, the student will be able to perform the following:

- Identify and document important information that should be included in your patient care report from a scene size-up.

- Choose the best format from different reporting styles for various patients with different types of medical and trauma conditions.

- Accurately and completely document subjective and objective findings from dispatch through various points in patient interactions, including initial assessments and interventions, as well as the rapid physical examination.

- Identify and apply reporting strategies you would use in special circumstances, such as calls when a crime may be involved.

- Demonstrate how you would document patient response to the delivery of incorrect care.

EXERCISE 1

 CD-ROM Activity

 Time: 15 minutes

- Sign into the software by entering your name in the name tag and clicking **Enter.**
- Choose the case by clicking on *Case 1: 20-year-old male—difficulty breathing.*
- Listen to the dispatch, or read it in the right panel (or both).
- Click **Start** and watch the entire video. Once the video has concluded, you are "on scene."
- Read the history log on the right side of the screen.
- You may use the **Look**, **Listen**, and **Feel** buttons, as well as determine pulse, blood pressure, and respiration readings before you answer the following question.

1. Begin the narrative in the following table using the CHART format. Provide the following information:

Aspect to Document	Answer
Chief complaint	
History	
Assessment	

- Click **Quit Case,** and you will be taken to the summary menu.

EXERCISE 2

 CD-ROM Activity

 Time: 15 minutes

2. Before you start the case, consider what you might observe at the scene of a crime involving a gunshot that would be considered important and should be included in the patient care report. List three observations.

   a.

   b.

   c.

- Click **Restart** from the summary menu.
- Choose the case by clicking on *Case 11: 32-year-old male—gunshot wounds.*
- Listen to the dispatch, or read it in the right panel (or both).
- Click **Start** and begin watching the video.
- Click **Pause (‖)** as soon as the shirt is cut and opened.

3. Using the chronologic call-incident or storytelling approach, write the first few sentences that would appear in your patient care narrative for this patient.

4. Describe how you would document in your patient care report the locations of the apparent bullet wounds you observed after opening the patient's shirt.

- Click **Play (▶)**. Once the video has concluded, you are "on scene."
- Read the history log on the right side of the screen.

5. Using the information gained, add these objective findings as you would document them in the narrative and vital signs areas in a patient care report.

 • Click **Quit Case,** and you will be taken to the summary menu.

EXERCISE 3

 CD-ROM Activity

 Time: 15 minutes

 • Click **Restart** from the summary menu.
• Choose the case by clicking on *Case 9: 22-year-old female—assault.*
• Listen to the dispatch, or read it in the right panel (or both).
• Click **Start** and begin watching the video.
• Click **Pause (❚❚)** when the officer, Sgt. Campbell, completes her briefing.

6. Recognizing that this case will likely go to court and that your patient care report will be evidence, consider what general observations about the patient's environment might be important and should be included in the patient care report. List two observations.

   a.

   b.

 • Click **Play (▶)** to resume the video.
• Click **Stop (■)** as soon as the patient finishes answering the question from the paramedic.

7. List several observations you would include in your report that would describe the apparent psychologic state of the patient with the expectation that you will present these observations in court.

8. You decide to perform a limited physical examination of the patient. How would your patient care report indicate the fact that you did not conduct a physical examination of the patient specific to the sexual assault?

- Click **Proceed**.
- Click **Quit Case,** and you will be taken to the summary menu.

EXERCISE 4

 CD-ROM Activity

 Time: 15 minutes

- Click **Restart** from the summary menu.
- Choose the case by clicking on *Case 14: 65-year-old male—difficulty breathing.*
- Listen to the dispatch, or read it in the right panel (or both).
- Click **Start** and begin watching the video.
- Click **Pause (II)** when the paramedic begins to tell the patient the dog is too loud.

9. This patient, when asked what was wrong, responded with two complaints. Which method of narrative reporting, SOAP or CHART, would work best in this case? Explain your answer.

- Click **Play (▶)**. Once the video has concluded, you are "on scene."
- Read the history log on the right side of the screen.

10. Complete the first part of your narrative using the SOAP format. List all the subjective data, skip a line, and then list all the objective data.

- Click **Quit Case,** and you will be taken to the summary menu.

EXERCISE 5

  CD-ROM Activity

 Time: 10 minutes

→
- Click **Restart** from the summary menu.
- Choose the case by clicking on *Case 13: 5-month-old male—unresponsive.*
- Listen to the dispatch, or read it in the right panel (or both).
- Click **Start** and watch the entire video. Once the video has concluded, you are "on scene."
- Read the history log on the right side of the screen.
- Using the **Assessment** buttons in the left panel, perform the initial assessment, including "looking" and "feeling," and begin treatment using only basic life support (BLS) skills such as oropharyngeal airways (OPAs) and cardiopulmonary resuscitation (CPR). Do not apply the monitor or defibrillator.

11. Keeping in mind that the parent has not accompanied you, what method of reporting will likely work best with this patient—SOAP, CHART, or the chronologic call-incident (storytelling) approach? Explain why your choice would be the best.

12. Begin your report using the chronologic call-incident or storytelling approach, beginning with your dispatch and continuing through the application of CPR using BLS equipment.

→
- Click **Quit Case,** and you will be taken to the summary menu.

EXERCISE 6

 CD-ROM Activity

 Time: 10 minutes

- Click **Restart** from the summary menu.
- Choose the case by clicking on *Case 8: 38-year-old male—suicide attempt*.
- Listen to the dispatch, or read it in the right panel (or both).
- Click **Start** and begin watching the video.
- Click Pause (**II**) when the police place the patient on the stretcher.

13. The police have secured this patient on the stretcher. You will need to document the restraint in your patient care report. List the appropriate dispatch information and your initial observations of the patient in a manner that justifies your decision to allow the police to gain control of the patient.

14. Because the police had to use force with this patient, some physical injuries may have resulted. Indicate how you would document the capturing, restraining, and moving of the patient to the stretcher by the police.

15. Describe how you would document the initial actions you would take after the police have positioned the patient on the stretcher and prepared him for transportation, including the actions you would take to reposition the patient appropriately.

- Click **Proceed**.
- Click **Quit Case,** and you will be taken to the summary menu.
- Click **Exit** to close the program, or **Restart** to continue with another lesson.

Head, Ear, Eye, Nose, and Throat Disorders

Reading Assignment: Read Chapter 20, Head, Ear, Eye, Nose, and Throat Disorders, in *Paramedic Practice Today: Above and Beyond.*

Case 12: 57-year-old male—man down.

Objectives:

On completion of this lesson, the student will be able to perform the following:

- When the patient has a chief complaint that includes "dizziness," determine whether the patient means vertigo or lightheadedness.
- Value the importance of distinguishing the difference between being lightheaded and having vertigo.

EXERCISE 1

 CD-ROM Activity

 Time: 15 minutes

- Sign into the software by entering your name in the name tag and clicking **Enter.**
- Choose the case by clicking on *Case 12: 57-year-old male—man down.*
- Listen to the dispatch, or read it in the right panel (or both).
- Click **Start** and watch the entire video. Once the video has concluded, you are "on scene."
- Read the history log on the right side of the screen.

1. What important additional question should you ask after the patient states that he was dizzy? What clinical impression or impressions would this information give you?

2. If this patient had reported that he had vertigo, what other clinical signs or symptoms might you expect to find? Where any of these clinical conditions present in this case?

- Click **Quit Case,** and you will be taken to the summary menu.
- Click **Exit** to close the program, or **Restart** to continue with another lesson.

Pulmonology

✎ **Reading Assignment:** Read Chapter 21, Pulmonology, in *Paramedic Practice Today: Above and Beyond*.

Other Relevant Chapters:
- Chapter 1, EMS Safety and Well-Being of the Paramedic
- Chapter 8, Pathophysiology
- Chapter 11, Basic Principles of Pharmacology
- Chapter 12, Drug and Chemical Classes
- Chapter 13, Medication Administration
- Chapter 16, History Taking
- Chapter 17, Patient Assessment
- Chapter 19, Documentation
- Chapter 31, Infectious and Communicable Diseases

Case 15: 42-year-old male—difficulty breathing

Objectives:

On completion of this lesson, the student will be able to perform the following:
- Form a clinical impression based on a careful history and physical examination.
- Identify key interventions needed to effect a favorable outcome for the patient.
- Recognize the appropriateness of safety interventions for emergency medical services (EMS) personnel in this case.

EXERCISE 1

 CD-ROM Activity

 Time: 15 minutes

- Sign into the software by entering your name in the name tag and clicking **Enter.**
- Choose the case by clicking on *Case 15: 42-year-old male—difficulty breathing.*
- Listen to the dispatch, or read it in the right panel (or both).
- Click **Start** and watch the entire video. Once the video has concluded, you are "on scene."
- Read the history log on the right side of the screen.
- Perform your assessments and interventions using the buttons in the left panel. When you have determined that it is appropriate to begin transporting your patient to the hospital, click the **Load Patient** button. Continue your assessments and interventions en route to the hospital. When you have finished treating your patient, click the **Unload Patient** button. You will be taken to the summary menu.
- Click the **Log** button on the summary menu, and review your patient care as you answer the following questions.

1. What is your clinical impression of this patient? Describe the historical and physical assessment cues that led you to that impression.

History	Physical Examination

2. What are your highest priorities for care for this patient?

3. What ECG rhythm did you observe? What is causing the rhythm? How will you manage it?

4. Explain why you selected the oxygen device and flow rate that you chose.

5. Was it appropriate for the prehospital providers to apply the masks? Explain your answer.

6. Describe the pathophysiologic cause of the signs and symptoms you observed in the patient as they relate to your clinical impression.

Sign or Symptom	Pathophysiologic Cause
Dyspnea	
Jugular venous distention (JVD)	
Decreased SaO_2	
Decreased $ETCO_2$	

7. The patient has tingling around his lips. Why do you think this sign is not hyperventilation related to an anxiety attack?

8. Distinguish the assessment findings for each of the following causes of respiratory distress. Then identify whether any of these findings are found in this patient.

Disease	Breath Sounds	History of Present Illness	Medical History	Capnography Waveform	Home Medicines (if history of the illness is known)
Pulmonary edema					
Found in this patient?					
Anaphylaxis					
Found in this patient?					
Pulmonary embolism					
Found in this patient?					

Disease	Breath Sounds	History of Present Illness	Medical History	Capnography Waveform	Home Medicines (if history of the illness is known)
Asthma					
Found in this patient?					
Pneumonia					
Found in this patient?					

9. Complete a patient care report (PCR) for this call. (Use one of the blank PCRs in the back of your study guide or one your instructor has given you.)

- To save your log, click on the disk icon. To print your log, click on the printer icon.
- Click **Menu** to return to the summary menu.
- Click **Exit** to close the program, or **Restart** to continue with another lesson.

EXERCISE 2

 Summary Activity

 Time: 15 minutes

10. How do you believe you handled this call?

11. Do you think you would change your actions if given the opportunity to complete the call again?

    If you said *yes,* what would you change and how do you think those changes would affect the patient?

 • Review your log with your instructor to see how it compares with the recommended care found in the *Implementation Manual.*

12. How did your care compare with what was recommended?

13. After reviewing the call, would you change anything on a subsequent call of this nature?

Cardiovascular Disorders I

Reading Assignment: Read Chapter 22, Cardiovascular Disorders, in *Paramedic Practice Today: Above and Beyond.*

Other Relevant Chapters:

- Chapter 8, Pathophysiology
- Chapter 11, Basic Principles of Pharmacology
- Chapter 12, Drug and Chemical Classes
- Chapter 13, Medication Administration
- Chapter 14, Airway Management
- Chapter 16, History Taking
- Chapter 17, Patient Assessment
- Chapter 19, Documentation
- Chapter 40, Patients with Special Challenges
- Chapter 56, Clinical Decision Making

Case 2: 56-year-old female—fell

Objectives:

On completion of this lesson, the student will be able to perform the following:

- Using an appropriate patient history and physical examination, establish the cause of the patient's illness.
- Deliver appropriate patient care in a sequence to maximize the patient's chance of recovery.
- Administer the appropriate drugs in the correct manner.
- Recognize and respond appropriately to changes in patient condition.
- Identify resources needed to appropriately care for an obese patient.

EXERCISE 1

 CD-ROM Activity

 Time: 15 minutes

➔
- Sign into the software by entering your name in the name tag and clicking **Enter.**
- Choose the case by clicking on *Case 2: 56-year-old female—fell.*
- Listen to the dispatch, or read it in the right panel (or both).
- Click **Start** and watch the entire video. Once the video has concluded, you are "on scene."

1. What was your impression of the patient when you saw the initial interview and images of her?

2. What was the initial ECG rhythm that you observed?

3. Do you think any relationship exists between the medications the patient is taking and the initial ECG rhythm? Explain the rationale for your answer.

4. What illnesses or injuries do you need to rule out, based on your initial impression of the patient?

5. Based on the medications the patient is taking, what medical history do you suspect in addition to the congestive heart failure (CHF) and cardiac problems that her husband reports?

Drug	Class	Prescription Use

6. What challenge related to transportation is evident in the initial video images of this patient?

7. Describe strategies that you might use to manage the challenges that you identified.

EXERCISE 2

 CD-ROM Activity

 Time: 15 minutes

- Read the history log on the right side of the screen.
- Perform your assessments and interventions using the buttons in the left panel. When you have determined that it is appropriate to begin transporting your patient to the hospital, click the **Load Patient** button. Continue your assessments and interventions en route to the hospital. When you have finished treating your patient, click the **Unload Patient** button. You will be taken to the summary menu.
- Click the **Log** button on the summary menu, and review your patient care as you answer the following questions.

8. Assume that you obtained a 12-lead ECG before the patient's condition changed and that it appears as follows:

a. Describe your interpretation of this ECG.

b. What actions should you take, based on these findings?

9. Compare the following characteristics of biphasic versus monophasic defibrillators.

	Monophasic Defibrillator	Biphasic Defibrillator
Energy level used to treat ventricular fibrillation for first defibrillation, if manufacturer's recommendations are unknown		
Second and subsequent defibrillation energy level, if manufacturer recommendations are unknown		
Current is delivered using pads or paddles?		
Adjusts current delivered based on chest impedence before shock delivery?	*(Yes or No)*	*(Yes or No)*

10. After you place the endotracheal tube, you observe the following findings. State what these assessment findings indicate and the actions you would take.

Finding	Indicates	Actions Needed
a. Esophageal detector device bulb fills in less than 2 seconds.		
b. Breath sounds are audible over the left lung but absent over the right lung.		
c. Capnography waveform is observed.		
d. The end-tidal carbon dioxide ($ETCO_2$) detector alternates in color between purple and yellow after the sixth ventilation.		

11. For each drug you administered in this case, indicate the volume of the drug that you administered and at least one desired effect of that drug.

Drug and Dose	Volume Given	Desired Effect

Drug and Dose	Volume Given	Desired Effect

12. Would terminating resuscitation be appropriate in this case?

   If you answered *yes,* then describe at what point in the resuscitation it would be appropriate.

   If you answered *no*, then describe why this patient would not be an appropriate candidate for this decision.

13. Complete a patient care report (PCR) for this call. (Use one of the blank PCRs in the back of your study guide or the one your instructor has given you.)

→ • To save your log, click on the disk icon. To print your log, click on the printer icon.
   • Click **Menu** to return to the summary menu.
   • Click **Exit** to close the program, or **Restart** to continue with another lesson.

EXERCISE 3

 Summary Activity

 Time: 15 minutes

14. How do you feel about how you handled this call?

15. Do you think you would change your actions if given the opportunity to complete the call again?

    If you said *yes,* what would you change and how do you think those changes would affect the patient?

 • Review your log with your instructor to see how it compares with the recommended care found in the *Implementation Manual*.

16. How did your care compare with what was recommended?

17. After reviewing the call, would you change anything on a subsequent call of this kind?

 • Click **Quit Case,** and you will be taken to the summary menu.
• Click **Exit** to close the program, or **Restart** to continue with another lesson.

Cardiovascular Disorders II

Reading Assignment: Read Chapter 22, Cardiovascular Disorders, in *Paramedic Practice Today: Above and Beyond*.

Other Relevant Chapters:

- Chapter 8, Pathophysiology
- Chapter 11, Basic Principles of Pharmacology
- Chapter 12, Drug and Chemical Classes
- Chapter 14, Airway Management
- Chapter 17, Patient Assessment
- Chapter 19, Documentation
- Chapter 22, Pulmonology

Case 14: 65-year-old male—difficulty breathing

Objectives:

On completion of this lesson, the student will be able to perform the following:

- Distinguish cardiac from noncardiac causes of dyspnea.
- Perform appropriate interventions for the patient with dyspnea, based on appropriate pathophysiologic knowledge.

EXERCISE 1

 CD-ROM Activity

 Time: 15 minutes

- Sign into the software by entering your name in the name tag and clicking **Enter.**
- Choose the case by clicking on *Case 14: 65-year-old male—difficulty breathing.*
- Listen to the dispatch, or read it in the right panel (or both).
- Click **Start** and watch the entire video. Once the video has concluded, you are "on scene."
- Read the history log on the right side of the screen.
- Perform your assessments and interventions using the buttons in the left panel. When you have determined that it is appropriate to begin transporting your patient to the hospital, click the **Load Patient** button. Continue your assessments and interventions en route to the hospital. When you have finished treating your patient, click the **Unload Patient** button. You will be taken to the summary menu.
- Click the **Log** button on the summary menu and review your patient care as you answer the following questions.

1. While watching the video, did you observe anything in the background of the situation? How could your observations influence your call? What actions might you need to take to address this situation?

2. What was the significance of the patient's home oxygen?

3. List the classification and indications for each of the home medicines this patient takes.

Medicine	Classification	Indications	Side Effects

4. What is your clinical impression of this patient? Describe the factors that led you to this determination.

5. Assume you had the capability to perform a 12-lead ECG examination and you obtained the following rhythm. Describe your interpretation of the rhythm and whether it is consistent with this patient's clinical picture.

6. Describe each drug you used to treat this patient and the desired mechanism of action.

Drug	Rationale
Aspirin	
Nitroglycerin	
Morphine	
Furosemide	

7. List nonpharmacologic interventions for this patient and your rationale for using them.

8. For each of the physical findings listed in the following table, describe how you would assess it and the pathophysiologic significance of each finding.

Finding	Assessment Technique	Significance
Crackles in the lungs		
Jugular venous distention		
Pedal edema		

9. Explain how the use of capnography might influence your treatment decisions for this patient.

10. Complete a patient care report (PCR) for this call. (Use one of the blank PCRs in the back of your study guide or one your instructor has given you.)

→ • To save your log, click on the disk icon. To print your log, click on the printer icon.
   • Click **Menu** to return to the summary menu.
   • Click **Exit** to close the program, or **Restart** to continue with another lesson.

EXERCISE 2

Summary Activity

Time: 15 minutes

11. How did you feel about how you handled this call?

12. Do you think you would change your actions if given the opportunity to complete the call again?

    If you said *yes,* what would you change and how do you think those changes would affect the patient?

 • Review your log with your instructor to see how it compares with the recommended care found in the *Implementation Manual.*

13. How did your care compare with what was recommended?

14. After reviewing the call, would you change anything on a subsequent call of this nature?

Disorders of the Nervous System

👓 **Reading Assignment:** Read Chapter 23, Disorders of the Nervous System, in *Paramedic Practice Today: Above and Beyond*.

Other Relevant Chapters:
- Chapter 1, EMS Safety and Well-Being of the Paramedic
- Chapter 8, Pathophysiology
- Chapter 9, Life Span Development
- Chapter 11, Basic Principles of Pharmacology
- Chapter 12, Drug and Chemical Classes
- Chapter 13, Medication Administration
- Chapter 14, Airway Management
- Chapter 15, Therapeutic Communication
- Chapter 17, Patient Assessment
- Chapter 31, Infectious and Communicable Diseases
- Chapter 37, Pediatrics
- Chapter 39, Abuse and Assault

Case 3: 7-year-old female—seizure

Objectives:

On completion of this lesson, the student will be able to perform the following:
- Describe the rationale for specific scene safety considerations on this call.
- Perform appropriate patient assessments in the correct sequence.
- Interpret signs and symptoms based on knowledge of pathophysiology to develop a clinical impression.
- Indicate appropriate patient management strategies.
- Evaluate the effectiveness of patient interventions.
- Document the call appropriately.

EXERCISE 1

 CD-ROM Activity

 Time: 15 minutes

- Sign into the software by entering your name in the name tag and clicking **Enter.**
- Choose the case by clicking on *Case 3: 7-year-old female—seizure.*
- Listen to the dispatch, or read it in the right panel (or both).

1. What clinical conditions come to mind based on the dispatch information only?

2. Would the age of the patient influence your previous answer?

- Click **Start** and watch the entire video. Once the video has concluded, you are "on scene."
- Read the history log on the right side of the screen.
- Perform your assessments and interventions using the buttons in the left panel. When you have determined that it is appropriate to begin transporting your patient to the hospital, click the **Load Patient** button. Continue your assessments and interventions en route to the hospital. When you have finished treating your patient, click the **Unload Patient** button. You will be taken to the summary menu.
- Click the **Log** button on the summary menu, and review your patient care as you answer the following questions.

3. What ECG rhythm did you observe? What could be causing this rhythm in this patient?

4. Explain why you performed the airway interventions you selected.

5. Describe the rationale for safety interventions that the crews used on this call.

6. What are some possible explanations for the child's father's behavior?

7. What illness or injury do you believe has caused this child's signs and symptoms?

8. Describe the characteristics of petechiae.

9. This child had petechiae on her trunk and extremities. How might your clinical impression have changed if the petechiae were on her head and face only?

10. Describe the characteristics of this child that make her susceptible to abuse.

11. Under what circumstances would it be necessary for you to be placed on postexposure prophylaxis related to this call?

12. Describe your rationale for selecting the particular fluid administration type and volume for this patient.

13. Distinguish the characteristics of absence (petit mal), simple partial, complex partial, and tonic-clonic (grand mal) seizures. Discuss whether this child's signs and symptoms fit each category.

Seizure Type	Specific or Generalized Focus?	Signs and Symptoms	Age Specific?	How Does This Patient Fit Characteristics?
Absence (petit mal)				
Simple partial				
Complex partial				
Tonic-clonic (grand mal)				

14. Indicate two alternatives to the drug that you administered to treat this patient's seizures (include the dose and rate of intravenous [IV] administration). Indicate whether this drug could be given by another route (if vascular access was not possible).

Drug	Dose	Rate	Alternate Route?

15. Based on your related knowledge of the patient's illness, what should you tell the patient's mother when she asks you whether her child is "going to be okay"?

16. Graph the systolic blood pressure (BP) and heart rate that you obtained in this call (consult your log), then connect the data points so that each vital sign forms a line (see example). You can use blue ink for the systolic BP and red ink for the heart rate.

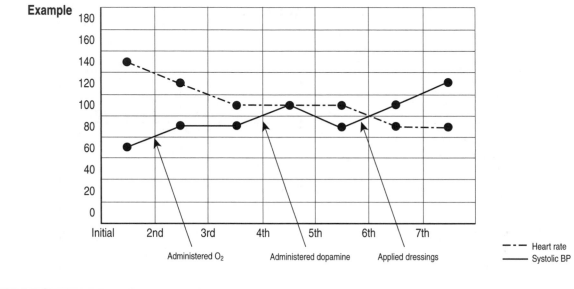

17. Referring to your own graph on the previous page, answer the following questions:

    a. What trends do you observe?

    b. How did your interventions relate to the trends you observe? (You may want to label your graph with interventions performed at various intervals as shown on the example.)

    c. If the trend reversed at any point, how can you explain that variation?

18. Complete a patient care report (PCR) for this call. (Use one of the blank PCRs in the back of your study guide or the one your instructor has given you.)

 • To save your log, click on the disk icon. To print your log, click on the printer icon.

     • Click **Menu** to return to the summary menu.

     • Click **Exit** to close the program, or **Restart** to continue with another lesson.

EXERCISE 2

Summary Activity

Time: 15 minutes

19. How do you feel about how you handled this call?

20. Do you think you would change your actions if given the opportunity to complete the call again?

    If you said *yes,* what would you change and how do you think those changes would affect the patient?

 • Review your log with your instructor to see how it compares the the recommended care found in the *Implementation Manual.*

21. How did your care compare with what was recommended?

22. After reviewing the call, would you change anything on a subsequent call of this kind?

Endocrine Emergencies and Nutritional Disorders

✏️ **Reading Assignment:** Read Chapter 24, Endocrine Emergencies and Nutritional Disorders, in *Paramedic Practice Today: Above and Beyond.*

Other Relevant Chapters:

- Chapter 8, Pathophysiology
- Chapter 11, Basic Principles of Pharmacology
- Chapter 12, Drug and Chemical Classes
- Chapter 13, Medication Administration
- Chapter 16, History Taking
- Chapter 17, Patient Assessment
- Chapter 23, Disorders of the Nervous System
- Chapter 38, Geriatrics

Case 4: 64-year-old male—unknown medical

Objectives:

On completion of this lesson, the student will be able to perform the following:

- Distinguish among key signs and symptoms to form a clinical impression of a patient with altered level of consciousness.
- Identify appropriate interventions for the patient with altered level of consciousness.
- Perform assessment and reassessment in the appropriate sequence.
- Document the call appropriately.

EXERCISE 1

 CD-ROM Activity

 Time: 15 minutes

- Sign into the software by entering your name in the name tag and clicking **Enter.**
- Choose the case by clicking on *Case 4: 64-year-old male—unknown medical.*
- Listen to the dispatch, or read it in the right panel (or both).
- Click **Start** and watch the entire video. Once the video has concluded, you are "on scene."

1. Based on the dispatcher's information, initial scene observations, and the family's observations, state at least five differential diagnoses that you need to rule out. Describe your rationale for each.

Possible Diagnosis	Rationale
1.	
2.	
3.	
4.	
5.	

- Read the history log on the right side of the screen.
- Perform your assessments and interventions using the buttons in the left panel. When you have determined that it is appropriate to begin transporting your patient to the hospital, click the **Load Patient** button. Continue your assessments and interventions en route to the hospital. When you have finished treating your patient, click the **Unload Patient** button. You will be taken to the summary menu.
- Click the **Log** button on the summary menu, and review your patient care as you answer the following questions.

2. What additional assessments did you need to perform to rule out stroke?

3. Explain how you would perform these assessments in real life.

4. If you think the patient is having a stroke, would you still treat his hypoglycemia in the same manner?

   If you said *no*, then explain your answer.

5. If you think the patient is having a stroke, what information would be essential for the hospital to know?

6. Would a high index of suspicion for stroke influence your decision regarding where to transport the patient?

If you said *yes,* then explain your answer.

7. Respond to the following questions, based on the fact that the patient is taking an oral hypoglycemic agent:

a. What additional questions should you ask the patient?

b. Would the care you administer change?

c. Would the information given to the patient change if the patient refuses care?

8. If you elected to administer oral medication to this patient, then describe actions that you should take before giving it, to ensure patient safety.

9. Describe the pathophysiologic basis for the signs and symptoms you observed in the patient on this call.

Sign or Symptom	Pathophysiologic Basis
Diaphoresis	
Altered mental status	
Tachycardia	

10. What age-related factors increase this patient's risk for complications related to diabetes?

11. Complete a patient care report (PCR) for this call. (Use one of the blank PCRs in the back of your study guide or the one your instructor has given you.)

 • To save your log, click on the disk icon. To print your log, click on the printer icon.
  • Click **Menu** to return to the summary menu.
  • Click **Exit** to close the program, or **Restart** to continue with another lesson.

EXERCISE 2

Summary Activity

Time: 15 minutes

12. How do you feel about the way you handled this call?

13. Do you think you would change your actions if given the opportunity to complete the call again?

    If you said *yes,* what would you change and how do you think those changes would affect the patient?

- Review your log with your instructor to see how it compares the the recommended care found in the *Implementation Manual.*

14. How did your care compare with what was recommended?

15. After reviewing the call, would you change anything on a subsequent call of this kind?

Immune System Disorders

📖 **Reading Assignment:** Read Chapter 25, Immune System Disorders, in *Paramedic Practice Today: Above and Beyond*.

Other Relevant Chapters:
- Chapter 7, Body Systems: Anatomy and Physiology
- Chapter 8, Pathophysiology
- Chapter 11, Basic Priniciples of Pharmacology
- Chapter 12, Drug and Chemical Classes
- Chapter 13, Medication Administration
- Chapter 14, Airway Management
- Chapter 16, History Taking
- Chapter 17, Patient Assessment
- Chapter 18, Communications
- Chapter 19, Documentation
- Chapter 52, Environmental Conditions

Case 1: 20-year-old male—difficulty breathing

Objectives:

On completion of this lesson, the student will be able to perform the following:
- Establish the cause of the patient's difficulty breathing using an appropriate patient history and physical examination.
- Deliver appropriate patient care in a sequence to maximize the patient's chance of recovery.
- Administer the appropriate drugs in the correct manner.
- Document the call appropriately.

EXERCISE 1

 CD-ROM Activity

 Time: 15 minutes

- Sign into the software by entering your name in the name tag and clicking **Enter.**
- Choose the case by clicking on *Case 1: 20-year-old male—difficulty breathing.*
- Listen to the dispatch, or read it in the right panel (or both).
- Click **Start** and watch the entire video. Once the video has concluded, you are "on scene."

1. What information would lead the dispatcher to state that the cause of the breathing problem is related to an allergic reaction?

2. During your initial observation of the scene, what do you notice that might create some difficulty if the patient is transported?

3. Do the signs and symptoms reported by the emergency medical responders indicate that administration of epinephrine was appropriate?

   If you said *yes,* list the specific findings that justify your answer.

4. How long must you wait before administering a second dose of epinephrine if it is indicated?

• Read the history log on the right side of the screen.

- Perform your assessments and interventions using the buttons in the left panel. When you have determined that it is appropriate to begin transporting your patient to the hospital, click the **Load Patient** button. Continue your assessments and interventions en route to the hospital. When you have finished treating your patient, click the **Unload Patient** button. You will be taken to the summary menu.

- Click the **Log** button on the summary menu, and review your patient care as you answer the following questions.

5. What was the initial ECG rhythm you observed?

6. Why would the patient have this rhythm?

7. Explain your rationale for selecting the particular oxygen device and flow rate you selected for this patient.

8. What additional physical findings for this patient confirm your clinical impression?

9. Describe how the chemical mediators released in anaphylaxis caused the signs and symptoms you observed in the patient on this call.

Chemical Mediator	Pathophysiologic Effect	Associated Sign or Symptom
Histamine		
Leukotrienes		

10. Explain why epinephrine, in the appropriate dose and route, will improve this patient's condition.

11. If an excessive dose of epinephrine were to be given, describe the possible effect it might have on this patient.

12. If the administration of intravenous (IV) epinephrine was needed in this case, complete the following information related to its administration:

  a. Dose:

  b. Concentration:

  c. Rate of administration:

13. If the only drug you administered was albuterol, would it resolve the patient's signs and symptoms? Justify your response.

14. Explain why this patient needs an infusion of IV fluids.

15. Describe how your approach to care would change if this patient were a 9-year-old, 40-kg child.

a. Drug doses:

b. IV fluid infusion:

16. For each drug that you administered in this case, describe at least two side effects that you should anticipate.

Drug	Dose	Route	Side Effects

17. Graph the systolic blood pressure (BP) and heart rate that you obtained in this call (consult your log); then connect the data points so that each vital sign forms a line (see example). You can use blue ink for the systolic BP and red ink for the heart rate.

18. Referring to your own graph on the previous page, answer the following questions:

a. What trends do you observe?

b. How did your interventions relate to the trends you observe? (You may want to label your graph with interventions performed at various intervals as shown on the example.)

c. If the trend reversed at any point, how can you explain that variation?

19. Complete a patient care report (PCR) for this call. (Use one of the blank PCRs in the back of your study guide or the one your instructor has given you.)

➤ • To save your log, click on the disk icon. To print your log, click on the printer icon.
   • Click **Menu** to return to the summary menu.
   • Click **Exit** to close the program, or **Restart** to continue with another lesson.

EXERCISE 2

 Summary Activity

 Time: 15 minutes

20. How do you feel about how you handled this call?

21. Do you think you would change your actions if given the opportunity to complete the call again?

    If you said *yes,* what would you change, and how do you think your changes would affect the patient?

 • Review your log with your instructor to see how it compares the the recommended care found in the *Implementation Manual.*

22. How did your care compare with what was recommended?

23. After reviewing the call, would you change anything on a subsequent call of this kind?

LESSON 28

Gastrointestinal Disorders

Reading Assignment: Read Chapter 26, Gastrointestinal Disorders, in *Paramedic Practice Today: Above and Beyond*.

Other Relevant Chapters:

- Chapter 1, EMS Safety and Well-Being of the Paramedic
- Chapter 8, Pathophysiology
- Chapter 14, Airway Management
- Chapter 16, History Taking
- Chapter 30, Toxicology
- Chapter 56, Clinical Decision Making

Case 5: 40-year-old male—vomiting blood

Objectives:

On completion of this lesson, the student will be able to perform the following:

- Perform an appropriate patient history and physical examination to establish clinical priorities of care.
- Establish a list of differential diagnoses based on the clinical findings present in this case.
- Deliver appropriate patient care in a sequence to maximize the patient's chance of recovery.
- Identify appropriate interventions for the patient who is vomiting blood.
- Anticipate appropriate personal protective equipment (PPE) that would be needed on a call with a patient who is vomiting blood.
- Document the call appropriately.

167

EXERCISE 1

 CD-ROM Activity

 Time: 15 minutes

- Sign into the software by entering your name in the name tag and clicking **Enter**.
- Choose the case by clicking on *Case 5: 40-year-old male—vomiting blood*.
- Listen to the dispatch, or read it in the right panel (or both).
- Click **Start** and watch the entire video. Once the video has concluded, you are "on scene."
- Read the history log on the right side of the screen.
- Perform your assessments and interventions using the buttons in the left panel. When you have determined that it is appropriate to begin transporting your patient to the hospital, click the **Load Patient** button. Continue your assessments and interventions en route to the hospital. When you have finished treating your patient, click the **Unload Patient** button. You will be taken to the summary menu.
- Click the **Log** button on the summary menu, and review your patient care as you answer the following questions.

1. Explain why you selected the particular oxygen device and flow rate.

2. What safety measures should you and your partner take based on your initial impression of the patient?

3. What airway equipment should you have ready after you perform your initial assessment? Explain your rationale.

4. In what position would you transport this patient? Explain your rationale.

5. List the differential diagnosis (or diagnoses) you should consider in this case based on the following clinical findings. You may select more than one.

Findings	Clinical Impression
Abdominal pain	
Vomiting bright-red blood	
Antibiotic therapy for 10 days	
History of gastroenteritis	
Vomits often	
Pain associated with drinking	
Intense, nonradiating pain	

6. What information related to the case might lead you to believe that this patient is an alcoholic?

7. How does chronic drinking increase a person's risk for gastrointestinal bleeding?

8. If you measured the patient's blood glucose at 40 mg/dL, you would administer dextrose 50% ($D_{50}W$). Based on this patient's history, what drug should be given with the dextrose (include dose and route)?

9. Explain why this drug is needed and the possible consequences should you not administer it.

10. Identify the advantages and disadvantages of these fluids as they relate to resuscitating this patient.

Fluid	Advantages for Use in This Case	Disadvantages for Use in This Case
0.9% Normal saline or Ringer's lactate		
0.45% Normal saline		
Whole blood		
Blood plasma		

11. List at least two disadvantages of large-volume crystalloid fluid resuscitation.

12. Explain whether dopamine would be the first choice to restore cardiac output in this patient.

13. Why would a patient with a history of chronic alcoholism be less able to compensate if bleeding and shock develop?

14. Complete a patient care report (PCR) for this call. (Use one of the blank PCRs in the back of your study guide or the one your instructor has given you.)

- To save your log, click on the disk icon. To print your log, click on the printer icon.
- Click **Menu** to return to the summary menu.
- Click **Exit** to close the program, or **Restart** to continue with another lesson.

EXERCISE 2

Summary Activity

Time: 15 minutes

15. How do you feel about how you handled this call?

16. Do you think you would change your actions if given the opportunity to complete the call again?

If you said *yes,* what would you change and how do you think those changes would affect the patient?

• Review your log with your instructor to see how it compares with the recommended care found in the *Implementation Manual*.

17. How did your care compare with what was recommended?

18. After reviewing the call, would you change anything on a subsequent call of this kind?

Renal and Urogenital Disorders

_____

Reading Assignment: Read Chapter 27, Renal and Urogenital Disorders, in *Paramedic Practice Today: Above and Beyond.*

Case 14: 65-year-old male—difficulty breathing

Objectives:

On completion of this lesson, the student will be able to perform the following:

- Anticipate complications of renal failure that can affect patient care.
- Describe appropriate assessment and management of the patient with renal failure.

EXERCISE 1

 CD-ROM Activity

 Time: 10 minutes

- Sign into the software by entering your name in the name tag and clicking **Enter.**
- Choose the case by clicking on *Case 14: 65-year-old male—difficulty breathing.*
- Listen to the dispatch, or read it in the right panel (or both).
- Click **Start** and watch the entire video. Once the video has concluded, you are "on scene."
- Read the history log on the right side of the screen.

Assume that, in this case, the patient tells you that he was recently diagnosed with renal failure. He has a shunt in his right forearm and had a trial of dialysis 2 weeks earlier, but he missed this week's appointment.

1. How does this information affect your clinical impression of the patient?

2. Describe any modification in patient assessment that you must take when caring for this patient.

3. How does renal failure affect the oxygen-carrying capacity of the blood?

4. Assume that your patient has the following ECG rhythm. His blood pressure is 70/50 mm Hg, and he has crackles throughout his lungs.

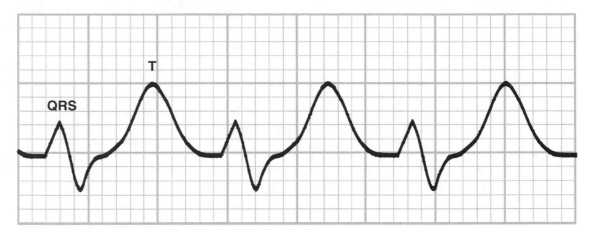

   a. In what position will you transport the patient? Explain your answer.

   b. Interpret the ECG.

5. What variations in the following laboratory values should you anticipate?

Laboratory Values	Anticipated Variations
pH	
Potassium	

Laboratory Values	Anticipated Variations
Lactic acid	
Blood urea nitrogen	
Creatinine	

6. The patient tells you his physician called yesterday and said that he had a high level of potassium. He immediately went into cardiac arrest. You note asystole on the monitor. List the sequence of drugs you will administer to this patient. Explain your rationale for each drug.

Drug	Rationale

7. Had the patient not been in arrest, what additional drug could be of benefit for hyperkalemia?

 • Click **Quit Case,** and you will be taken to the summary menu.
• Click **Exit** to close the program, or **Restart** to continue with another lesson.

Toxicology

Reading Assignment: Read Chapter 30, Toxicology, in *Paramedic Practice Today: Above and Beyond*.

Other Relevant Chapters:
- Chapter 8, Pathophysiology
- Chapter 11, Basic Principles of Pharmacology
- Chapter 12, Drug and Chemical Classes
- Chapter 13, Medication Administration
- Chapter 14, Airway Management
- Chapter 16, History Taking
- Chapter 17, Patient Assessment
- Chapter 22, Cardiovascular Disorders
- Chapter 23, Disorders of the Nervous System
- Chapter 32, Psychiatric Disorders and Substance Abuse

Case 6: 16-year-old female—unknown medical

Objectives:

On completion of this lesson, the student will be able to perform the following:
- Identify priorities of care in an unresponsive patient based on a thorough patient assessment.
- Interpret signs and symptoms based on knowledge of pathophysiology to develop a clinical impression.
- Indicate appropriate patient management strategies.
- Evaluate the effectiveness of patient interventions.
- Document the call appropriately.

EXERCISE 1

  CD-ROM Activity

 Time: 15 minutes

- Sign into the software by entering your name in the name tag and clicking **Enter.**
- Choose the case by clicking on *Case 6: 16-year-old female—unknown medical.*
- Listen to the dispatch, or read it in the right panel (or both).
- Click **Start** and watch the entire video. Once the video has concluded, you are "on scene."
- Read the history log on the right side of the screen.
- Perform your assessments and interventions using the buttons in the left panel. When you have determined that it is appropriate to begin transporting your patient to the hospital, click the **Load Patient** button. Continue your assessments and interventions en route to the hospital. When you have finished treating your patient, click the **Unload Patient** button. You will be taken to the summary menu.
- Click the **Log** button on the summary menu, and review your patient care as you answer the following questions.

1. What ECG rhythm did you observe?

2. Why is this rhythm a significant finding in this patient?

3. Predict how the ECG rhythm might change if the patient is not treated appropriately.

4. Explain your choice of airway-ventilation-oxygenation device.

5. Given the same initial vital signs (except respiratory rate) observed in this case, select the appropriate airway-oxygenation-ventilation delivery method based on the following capnographic findings. Explain why you chose this device.

Capnography Reading (Waveform)	Appropriate Oxygen Delivery Device	Rationale

6. If the patient is anorexic, what electrolyte abnormalities might she have? Could any of these explain the signs and symptoms she is experiencing? Explain your rationale.

7. List the drug class and indications for the use of Elavil.

8. Explain why ingestion of an excessive amount of Elavil could cause the signs and symptoms you observed in the patient on this call.

Sign or Symptom	Explanation
Altered level of consciousness	
Fast heart rate	
Hypotension	

9. Describe three other mechanisms that might cause altered level of consciousness or unconsciousness in a patient who has taken an overdose.

(1)

(2)

(3)

10. For each drug that you administered in this case, list the class and describe the specific desired effect for this patient.

Drug	Class	Desired Effect

11. Graph the systolic blood pressure (BP) and heart rate that you obtained in this call (consult your log); then connect the data points so that each vital sign forms a line (see example). You can use blue ink for the systolic BP and red ink for the heart rate.

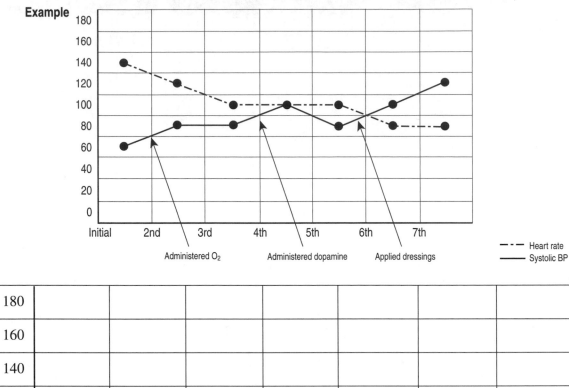

12. Referring to your own graph above, answer the following questions:

   a. What trends do you observe?

b. How did your interventions relate to the trends you observe? (You may want to label your graph with interventions performed at various intervals as shown on the example.)

c. If the trend reversed at any point, how can you explain that variation?

13. Complete a patient care report (PCR) for this call. (Use one of the blank PCRs in the back of your study guide or the one your instructor has given you.)

→
- To save your log, click on the disk icon. To print your log, click on the printer icon.
- Click **Menu** to return to the summary menu.
- Click **Exit** to close the program, or **Restart** to continue with another lesson.

EXERCISE 2

 Summary Activity

 Time: 15 minutes

14. How do you feel about how you handled this call?

15. Do you think you would change your actions if given the opportunity to complete the call again?

   If you said *yes,* what would you change and how do you think those changes would affect the patient?

 • Review your log with your instructor to see how it compares the recommended care found in the *Implementation Manual.*

16. How did your care compare with what was recommended?

17. After reviewing the call, would you change anything on a subsequent call of this kind?

Infectious and Communicable Diseases

✎ **Reading Assignment:** Read Chapter 31, Infectious and Communicable Diseases, in *Paramedic Practice Today: Above and Beyond.*

Case 15: 42-year-old male—difficulty breathing

Case 5: 40-year-old male—vomiting blood

Objectives:

On completion of this lesson, the student will be able to perform the following:

- Recognize appropriate personal protective equipment to prevent infectious disease exposure on selected cases.
- Outline how the chain of disease transmission relates to tuberculosis.
- Identify medications used to treat infectious diseases.
- Discuss actions that should be taken after exposure to blood or body fluids.

LESSON 31—INFECTIOUS AND COMMUNICABLE DISEASES

EXERCISE 1

 CD-ROM Activity

 Time: 15 minutes

- Sign into the software by entering your name in the name tag and clicking **Enter.**
- Choose the case by clicking on *Case 15: 42-year-old male—difficulty breathing.*
- Listen to the dispatch, or read it in the right panel (or both).
- Click **Start** and watch the entire video. Once the video has concluded, you are "on scene."
- Read the history log on the right side of the screen.

1. Explain how tuberculosis can be spread by identifying how its characteristics relate to each link in the chain of transmission of infection.

Link	Tuberculosis
Pathogenic agent	
Reservoir	
Portal of exit	
Transmission	
Portal of entry	
Host susceptibility	

Copyright © 2010 by Mosby, Inc., an affiliate of Elsevier Inc. All rights reserved.

2. If you suspect that a patient is infectious with pulmonary tuberculosis, what measures should you take to prevent exposure during the care and transport of this patient?

3. How should you clean the ambulance after the call?

4. Do you think this patient's acute signs and symptoms presented in this case are related to tuberculosis? Explain your answer.

5. Which of the patient's home medicines are used to treat tuberculosis?

6. List at least two other medications that may be used to treat tuberculosis.

7. If you were to be exposed to tuberculosis on this call and your purified protein derivative (PPD) skin test result in 6 months is positive, identify the following characteristics of prophylactic isoniazid, the drug you will likely take to prevent illness related to tuberculosis.

Drug	Should Avoid	Side Effects
Isoniazid		

 • Click **Quit Case,** and you will be taken to the summary menu.

EXERCISE 2

 CD-ROM Activity

 Time: 15 minutes

 • Click **Restart** from the summary menu.
• Choose the case by clicking on *Case 5: 40-year-old male—vomiting blood.*
• Listen to the dispatch, or read it in the right panel (or both).
• Click **Start** and watch the entire video. Once the video has concluded, you are "on scene."
• Read the history log on the right side of the screen.

8. What disease presents a high risk of exposure on this call?

9. What measures should the crew take to prevent significant exposure on this call?

10. Which of the following situations might represent a reportable significant exposure to blood or bloody body fluids on this call? What actions should you take before you report the exposure?

Situation	Significant? (Yes or No)	Immediate Actions Needed
Patient vomits, and you are certain that some of the vomit got into your eyes.		
A lancet barely pierces the skin on your thumb after assessing the level of blood glucose of the patient. You do not see any blood.		
When you arrive at the hospital, you notice some blood smeared on the intact skin of your forearm.		
While cleaning the ambulance after the call, an intravenous (IV) needle, which fell to the floor while this patient's IV was being started, sticks you. The wound is bleeding.		

11. Which of the significant exposures you identified in the previous question presents the highest risk?

12. What history or physical findings would identify a patient as being at particularly high risk for an infectious disease?

13. Answer the following questions related to follow-up if you had a significant exposure on this call.

    a. To whom should you report this exposure?

    b. When should you report this exposure?

14. Identify the specific postexposure prophylaxis (PEP) that is available for each of the following infectious diseases?

Disease	Postexposure Prophylaxis
Human immunodeficiency virus	
Hepatitis B (HBV)	
Hepatitis C (HCV)	

 • Click **Quit Case,** and you will be taken to the summary menu.
    • Click **Exit** to close the program, or **Restart** to continue with another lesson.

Psychiatric Disorders and Substance Abuse

/OTO **Reading Assignment:** Read Chapter 32, Psychiatric Disorders and Substance Abuse, in
Paramedic Practice Today: Above and Beyond.

Other Relevant Chapters:

- Chapter 1, EMS Safety and Well-Being of the Paramedic
- Chapter 4, Legal and Regulatory Issues
- Chapter 5, Ethics
- Chapter 11, Basic Principles of Pharmacology
- Chapter 12, Drug and Chemical Classes
- Chapter 13, Medication Administration
- Chapter 14, Airway Management
- Chapter 16, History Taking
- Chapter 17, Patient Assessment
- Chapter 19, Documentation

Case 8: 38-year-old male—suicide attempt

Objectives:

On completion of this lesson, the student will be able to perform the following:

- Demonstrate knowledge of the appropriate techniques to restrain a patient physically or chemically.
- Describe appropriate measures to monitor a restrained patient.
- Anticipate problems that can occur when a patient is restrained.
- Outline techniques to distinguish medical versus psychiatric causes of behavioral illness.
- Identify selected medications used to treat patients with behavioral illnesses.
- State appropriate techniques to use to communicate with a patient with a behavioral emergency.

EXERCISE 1

 CD-ROM Activity

 Time: 15 minutes

- Sign into the software by entering your name in the name tag and clicking **Enter.**
- Choose the case by clicking on *Case 8: 38-year-old male—suicide attempt*.
- Listen to the dispatch, or read it in the right panel (or both).
- Click **Start** and watch the entire video. Once the video has concluded, you are "on scene."
- Read the history log on the right side of the screen.
- Perform your assessments and interventions using the buttons in the left panel. When you have determined that it is appropriate to begin transporting your patient to the hospital, click the **Load Patient** button. Continue your assessments and interventions en route to the hospital. When you have finished treating your patient, click the **Unload Patient** button. You will be taken to the summary menu.
- Click the **Log** button on the summary menu, and review your patient care as you answer the following questions.

1. Why should you stage and not approach the scene on this type of dispatch until the police signal that the scene is safe?

2. How did the police place the patient on the stretcher?

3. Is leaving the patient restrained in that manner acceptable to you? Explain your answer.

4. Were the police officer's initial comments to the patient appropriate? Explain your answer.

5. What type of abnormal communication did you observe this patient make?

6. Could you predict at least two behavioral illnesses he might have? List three medications that he might be taking for each condition you listed and the side effect associated with each medication.

Behavioral Illness	Medications	Side Effects

7. During your assessment of this patient, you will need to rule out any organic cause of his bizarre behavior. List at least six possible organic causes of altered mental status and one or two specific signs or symptoms that you will assess to rule out these causes.

Organic Cause	Signs or Symptoms to Assess

8. List at least two alternate drugs that you could have administered in this case. Include the drug class, doses and routes of administration, and side effects you should anticipate. If the drug can be given intravenously (IV), then specify how fast you will administer it.

Drug	Class	Dose and Route	Possible Side Effects

9. What nonpharmacologic measures can you take to calm this patient's behavior during your care and transportation?

10. What specific patient assessment is necessary for a patient who is restrained?

11. Complete a patient care report (PCR) for this call. (Use one of the blank PCRs in the back of your study guide or one your instructor has given you.)

➡ • To save your log, click on the disk icon. To print your log, click on the printer icon.
   • Click **Menu** to return to the summary menu.
   • Click **Exit** to close the program, or **Restart** to continue with another lesson.

EXERCISE 2

 Summary Activity

Time: 10 minutes

12. How do you believe you handled this call?

13. Do you think you would change your actions if given the opportunity to complete the call again?

    If you said *yes*, what would you change and how do you think those changes would affect the patient?

• Review your log with your instructor to see how it compares with the recommended care found in the *Implementation Manual*.

14. How did your care compare with what was recommended?

15. After reviewing the call, would you change anything on a subsequent call of this nature?

Hematologic Disorders

👓 **Reading Assignment:** Read Chapter 33, Hematologic Disorders, in *Paramedic Practice Today: Above and Beyond.*

Case 15: 42-year-old male—difficulty breathing

Objectives:

On completion of this lesson, the student will be able to perform the following:

- Interpret this patient's signs and symptoms in the context of a history of sickle cell disease.
- Discuss the pathophysiologic characteristics of sickle cell disease.
- Identify interventions needed to manage the patient's signs and symptoms.

EXERCISE 1

 CD-ROM Activity

 Time: 10 minutes

- Sign into the software by entering your name in the name tag and clicking **Enter.**
- Choose the case by clicking on *Case 15: 42-year-old male—difficulty breathing.*
- Listen to the dispatch, or read it in the right panel (or both).
- Click **Start** and watch the entire video. Once the video has concluded, you are "on scene."
- Read the history log on the right side of the screen.

Assume that the patient tells you that he has sickle cell disease.

1. Could complications of sickle cell disease cause this patient's clinical presentation? Explain your answer.

2. What specific interventions should you perform for this patient if he has sickle cell disease?

3. Is the patient's history consistent with a situation that could cause sickle cell complications? Explain your answer.

4. Explain how sickle cell disease impairs his oxygen-carrying capacity before the onset of any acute illness.

5. Explain how the red blood cells respond if oxygen is not available to them.

6. List signs and symptoms, which may be present in a sickle cell crisis, that are related to cellular hypoxia.

7. If this patient's vacation were in a high-altitude region, could the altitude affect his sickle cell disease? Explain your answer.

  • Click **Quit Case,** and you will be taken to the summary menu.
  • Click **Exit** to close the program, or **Restart** to continue with another lesson.

Gynecology

Reading Assignment: Read Chapter 35, Obstetrics and Gynecology, in *Paramedic Practice Today: Above and Beyond*.

Case 9: 22-year-old female—assault

Case 6: 16-year-old female—unknown medical

Objectives:

On completion of this lesson, the student will be able to perform the following:

- Describe how an emotional response to a sexual assault can affect taking the patient's history.
- Identify gynecologic problems that can result in shock.
- Describe how to integrate evidence collection into the assessment and management of a patient who was sexually assaulted.

EXERCISE 1

 CD-ROM Activity

 Time: 15 minutes

- Sign into the software by entering your name in the name tag and clicking **Enter.**
- Choose the case by clicking on *Case 9: 22-year-old female—assault.*
- Listen to the dispatch, or read it in the right panel (or both).
- Click **Start** and watch the entire video. Once the video has concluded, you are "on scene."
- Read the history log on the right side of the screen.

1. Describe the patient's emotional response to the assault.

2. What other responses might you anticipate from a person who has been sexually assaulted?

3. How might you adapt your assessment and management of this patient to assist the patient emotionally?

4. List the priorities in the assessment and care of this patient.

5. What actions can you take or instruct the patient to take to preserve any evidence associated with the alleged assault?

6. How can you document your findings and the patient's statements to ensure that they will be legally defensible if introduced as evidence in the assault trial?

7. What injuries should you anticipate related to the sexual assault of a female patient?

 • Click **Quit Case,** and you will be taken to the summary menu.

EXERCISE 2

 CD-ROM Activity

 Time: 15 minutes

 • Click **Restart** from the summary menu.
- Choose the case by clicking on *Case 6: 16-year-old female—unknown medical.*
- Listen to the dispatch, or read it in the right panel (or both).
- Click **Start** and watch the entire video. Once the video has concluded, you are "on scene."
- Read the history log on the right side of the screen.
- Obtain one set of vital signs using the **Assessment** buttons in the left panel.

8. What gynecologic emergencies could cause this patient's signs and symptoms?

9. If this patient were conscious, what questions would you ask to determine whether a gynecologic problem is the cause of her emergency?

10. At what age do most women reach menarche?

11. Can you identify a possible reason why this patient may not yet have reached menarche?

➡ • Click **Quit Case,** and you will be taken to the summary menu.
 • Click **Exit** to close the program, or **Restart** to continue with another lesson.

Obstetrics

/ᴏᴏ **Reading Assignment:** Read Chapter 35, Obstetrics and Gynecology, in *Paramedic Practice Today: Above and Beyond.*

Other Relevant Chapters:
- Chapter 11, Basic Principles of Pharmacology
- Chapter 12, Drug and Chemical Classes
- Chapter 13, Medication Administration
- Chapter 14, Airway Management
- Chapter 15, Therapeutic Communication
- Chapter 16, History Taking
- Chapter 17, Patient Assessment
- Chapter 19, Documentation
- Chapter 23, Disorders of the Nervous System

Case 10: 25-year-old female—abdominal pain

Objectives:
On completion of this lesson, the student will be able to perform the following:
- Recognize and treat the complications of pregnancy.
- Anticipate signs and symptoms that may develop in a patient with complications of pregnancy.
- Demonstrate management of seizures in a pregnant patient.
- Anticipate the effects of interventions to manage complications of pregnancy.

EXERCISE 1

  CD-ROM Activity

 Time: 15 minutes

→
- Sign into the software by entering your name in the name tag and clicking **Enter.**
- Choose the case by clicking on *Case 10: 25-year-old female—abdominal pain.*
- Listen to the dispatch, or read it in the right panel (or both).
- Click **Start** and watch the entire video. Once the video has concluded, you are "on scene."
- Read the history log on the right side of the screen.
- Perform your assessments and interventions using the buttons in the left panel. When you have determined that it is appropriate to begin transporting your patient to the hospital, click the **Load Patient** button. Continue your assessments and interventions en route to the hospital. When you have finished treating your patient, click the **Unload Patient** button. You will be taken to the summary menu.
- Click the **Log** button on the summary menu, and review your patient care as you answer the following questions.

1. What communication barrier did you encounter on this call?

2. How would you have handled this barrier if the patient's friend were not present on the call?

3. Explain why you selected the oxygen device and flow rate that you did.

4. What additional physical findings might you observe that would confirm your initial clinical impression of this patient?

5. Describe the pathophysiologic causes of the signs and symptoms you observed in the patient on this call.

Sign or Symptom	Pathophysiologic Cause
Blood pressure (BP) 150/98 mm Hg	
Rash on abdomen	
Edema	

6. Transporting this patient involves important considerations.

   a. List two acceptable positions for this patient during transport:

b. Discuss measures that should be taken for supportive care of this patient during transport:

c. Describe how you might determine the appropriate transport destination for this patient:

7. This patient has severe abdominal pain.

a. What is a possible life-threatening cause of this pain?

b. For what signs and symptoms related to her pain will you assess?

c. What are the implications of the cause of this pain to the mother and fetus?

8. Describe how you might assess fetal heart tones (FHTs) on this patient.

9. You have assessed FHTs on this patient, and you observe the following findings. Discuss the significance of each finding.

Initial FHT	Significance
100 beats/min	
140 beats/min	
200 beats/min	

10. If this patient were to have a seizure, all of the benzodiazepines have a pregnancy category D.

    a. Describe what pregnancy category D means:

    b. Discuss how this category would affect your care:

11. List at least three drugs with appropriate doses and routes (including one that is not a benzodiazepine) that would be indicated to treat seizure activity in the patient.

Trade Name	Generic Name	Dose and Route

12. Complete a patient care report (PCR) for this call. (Use one of the blank PCRs in the back of your study guide or one your instructor has given you.)

→ • To save your log, click on the disk icon. To print your log, click on the printer icon.
   • Click **Menu** to return to the summary menu.
   • Click **Exit** to close the program, or **Restart** to continue with another lesson.

EXERCISE 2

 Summary Activity

 Time: 15 minutes

13. How do you believe you handled this call?

14. Do you think you would change your actions if given the opportunity to complete the call again?

If you said *yes,* what would you change and how do you think those changes would affect the patient?

• Review your log with your instructor to see how it compares with the recommended care found in the *Implementation Manual*.

15. How did your care compare with what was recommended?

16. After reviewing the call, would you change anything on a subsequent call of this kind?

Neonatology

/OZO **Reading Assignment:** Read Chapter 36, Neonatology, in *Paramedic Practice Today: Above and Beyond*.

Case 10: 25-year-old female—abdominal pain

Objectives:

On completion of this lesson, the student will be able to perform the following:

- Anticipate resuscitation measures that may be needed for a prehospital delivery.
- Describe an appropriate sequence of events during neonatal resuscitation that could lead to a favorable outcome.

EXERCISE 1

 CD-ROM Activity

 Time: 10 minutes

- Sign into the software by entering your name in the name tag and clicking **Enter.**
- Choose the case by clicking on *Case 10: 25-year-old female—abdominal pain.*
- Listen to the dispatch, or read it in the right panel (or both).
- Click **Start** and watch the entire video. Once the video has concluded, you are "on scene."
- Read the history log on the right side of the screen.
- Perform your initial assessment using the **Assessment** buttons in the left panel.

When you perform your assessment, assume that delivery is imminent, considering the initial history of this patient. You prepare to deliver this baby on the scene.

1. Based on the history that you have concerning this patient, explain whether you anticipate a high-risk delivery.

2. As the baby's head is delivered, you suction the airway. The shoulders then deliver quickly and you find yourself holding a floppy, blue baby. List your top four priorities at this time and the actions you will take to accomplish them.

Priorities	Actions

3. The baby is taking agonal gasps. Her heart rate is 50 beats/min. She is very pale.

   a. What could account for her condition?

   b. What are the immediate actions you need to take?

   c. If she does not respond favorably to your initial actions, what additional steps can you take?

4. Describe why intubation of this infant would be a high-risk procedure.

➤ • Click **Quit Case,** and you will be taken to the summary menu.
   • Click **Exit** to close the program, or **Restart** to continue with another lesson.

LESSON 37

Pediatrics I

📖 **Reading Assignment:** Read Chapter 37, Pediatrics, in *Paramedic Practice Today: Above and Beyond*.

Other Relevant Chapters:
- Chapter 3, Illness and Injury Prevention
- Chapter 8, Pathophysiology
- Chapter 14, Airway Management
- Chapter 17, Patient Assessment
- Chapter 48, Spinal Trauma

Case 7: 8-year-old male—submersion

Objectives:

On completion of this lesson, the student will be able to perform the following:

- Identify the priorities of patient care, based on an appropriate patient assessment.
- Predict potential injuries, based on the knowledge of mechanism of injury and relevant pathophysiologic characteristics.

EXERCISE 1

 CD-ROM Activity

 Time: 15 minutes

- Sign into the software by entering your name in the name tag and clicking **Enter.**
- Choose the case by clicking on *Case 7: 8-year-old male—submersion.*
- Listen to the dispatch, or read it in the right panel (or both).
- Click **Start** and watch the entire video. Once the video has concluded, you are "on scene."
- Read the history log on the right side of the screen.
- Perform your assessments and interventions using the buttons in the left panel. When you have determined that it is appropriate to begin transporting your patient to the hospital, click the **Load Patient** button. Continue your assessments and interventions en route to the hospital. When you have finished treating your patient, click the **Unload Patient** button. You will be taken to the summary menu.
- Click the **Log** button on the summary menu, and review your patient care as you answer the following questions.

1. The paramedics in this case approach a patient who was removed from the pool before their arrival. Are there safety considerations for this case if the patient has been removed from the water?

2. How should the patient be approached if he had remained in the water? What is the mnemonic for water rescue if the patient had been in a river or lake?

3. As the first responders approach, several errors are made. What are the errors and how would you correct them?

4. Detail the best way to manage this patient's airway.

5. Should nasotracheal intubation be attempted in this patient? Why?

6. The patient in this case is unconscious. List some differential diagnoses for possible reasons he might be unconscious.

7. The patient in this case had a near drowning incident in fresh water. Differentiate the pathophysiology of a fresh water and salt water drowning.

8. The lung sounds on auscultation are rhonchial. What would explain this?

9. The patient in this case was in warm water. Contrast the differences in a cold-water and warm-water drowning.

Cold-Water Drowning	Warm-Water Drowning

10. List signs and symptoms of hypothermia.

11. Prevention is often the key to avoiding a drowning incident. List some ideas for drowning prevention.

12. What is a "wet" drowning versus a "dry" drowning? Which of these most likely occurred with the patient in this case?

13. What pathophysiologic considerations should drive patient care and treatment in this case?

14. Complete a patient care report (PCR) for this call. (Use one of the blank PCRs in the back of your study guide or one your instructor has given you.)

→ • To save your log, click on the disk icon. To print your log, click on the printer icon.
  • Click **Menu** to return to the summary menu.
  • Click **Exit** to close the program, or **Restart** to continue with another lesson.

EXERCISE 2

Summary Activity

Time: 10 minutes

15. How do you believe you handled this call?

16. Do you think you would change your actions if given the opportunity to complete the call again?

    If you said *yes,* what would you change and how do you think those changes would affect the patient?

 • Review your log with your instructor to see how it compares with the recommended care found in the *Implementation Manual.*

17. How did your care compare with what was recommended?

18. After reviewing the call, would you change anything on a subsequent call of this nature? Explain your answer.

LESSON 38

Pediatrics II

ᴏ⃝ **Reading Assignment:** Read Chapter 37, Pediatrics, in *Paramedic Practice Today: Above and Beyond.*

Other Relevant Chapters:
- Chapter 3, Illness and Injury Prevention
- Chapter 4, Legal and Regulatory Issues
- Chapter 8, Pathophysiology
- Chapter 9, Life Span Development
- Chapter 11, Basic Principles of Pharmacology
- Chapter 13, Medication Administration
- Chapter 14, Airway Management
- Chapter 15, Therapeutic Communication
- Chapter 16, History Taking
- Chapter 17, Patient Assessment
- Chapter 19, Documentation
- Chapter 22, Cardiovascular Disorders
- Chapter 39, Abuse and Assault
- Chapter 40, Patients with Special Challenges

Case 13: 5-month-old male—unresponsive

Objectives:

On completion of this lesson, the student will be able to perform the following:
- Perform a rapid assessment to determine the priorities of care in a critically ill child.
- Prioritize patient interventions to deliver the most effective care in a critically ill child.
- Use effective communication techniques to obtain an accurate history and to facilitate a therapeutic relationship with the child's parents.

EXERCISE 1

 CD-ROM Activity

 Time: 15 minutes

- Sign into the software by entering your name in the name tag and clicking **Enter.**
- Choose the case by clicking on *Case 13: 5-month-old male—unresponsive.*
- Listen to the dispatch, or read it in the right panel (or both).
- Click **Start** and watch the entire video. Once the video has concluded, you are "on scene."
- Read the history log on the right side of the screen.
- Perform your assessments and interventions using the buttons in the left panel. When you have determined that it is appropriate to begin transporting your patient to the hospital, click the **Load Patient** button. Continue your assessments and interventions en route to the hospital. When you have finished treating your patient, click the **Unload Patient** button. You will be taken to the summary menu.
- Click the **Log** button on the summary menu, and review your patient care as you answer the following questions.

1. As the paramedics take the patient from the mother and move toward the ambulance, they instruct law enforcement to "please follow with mother." Are these directions appropriate? Why?

2. Use the pediatric assessment triangle and quickly assess this patient. Formulate your initial impression of this patient. Use the CUPS assessment scale to classify this patient.

3. What observations of the scene may have been useful if the paramedics had entered the residence?

4. List possible reasons for this child's cardiac arrest.

5. If first responders had been on location when the paramedics arrived, should an automatic external defibrillator have been placed on the patient? Why?

6. Calculate the endotracheal tube size for this child? Should the tube be cuffed or uncuffed? Why?

7. First responders have been on location in this case before arrival of the paramedics. During assessment, the paramedics note the abdomen is distended. Can this condition be corrected? List some ways to deal with this problem.

8. The paramedics in this case are unable to establish intravenous access. What is the next best option? Detail how you would establish this option.

9. What would the energy settings be for defibrillation and cardioversion of this child? How would those settings differ between a monophasic and a biphasic device?

10. What medications could be used during the resuscitation of this child? Calculate the dose based on the child's weight.

Medication	Pediatric Dose	Dose for This Child Child's Weight Is 7.3 kg

11. During transportation of the child in this lesson, it will be necessary to passively restrain the child. What are some ways to restrain the child for transport?

12. Complete a patient care report (PCR) for this call. (Use one of the blank PCRs in the back of your study guide or one your instructor has given you.)

- To save your log, click on the disk icon. To print your log, click on the printer icon.
- Click **Menu** to return to the summary menu.
- Click **Exit** to close the program, or **Restart** to continue with another lesson.

EXERCISE 2

Summary Activity

Time: 15 minutes

13. How did you feel about how you handled this call?

14. Do you think you would change your actions if given the opportunity to complete the call again?

If you said *yes,* what would you change and how do you think those changes would affect the patient?

• Review your log with your instructor to see how it compares with the recommended care found in the *Implementation Manual*.

15. How did your care compare with what was recommended?

16. After reviewing the call, would you change anything on a subsequent call of this nature?

Geriatrics

👓 **Reading Assignment:** Read Chapter 38, Geriatrics, in *Paramedic Practice Today: Above and Beyond..*

Other Relevant Chapters:
- Chapter 8, Pathophysiology
- Chapter 9, Life Span Development
- Chapter 15, Therapeutic Communication
- Chapter 16, History Taking
- Chapter 17, Patient Assessment

Case 14: 65-year-old male—difficulty breathing

Objectives:
On completion of this lesson, the student will be able to perform the following:
- Assess the living conditions and support for a geriatric patient.
- Communicate effectively with a geriatric patient during assessment.
- Assess and treat a geriatric patient.
- Address psychologic, emotional, and social needs during assessment of a geriatric patient.

EXERCISE 1

 CD-ROM Activity

 Time: 15 minutes

- Sign into the software by entering your name in the name tag and clicking **Enter**.
- Choose the case by clicking on *Case 14: 65-year-old male—difficulty breathing*.
- Listen to the dispatch, or read it in the right panel (or both).
- Click **Start** and watch the entire video. Once the video has concluded, you are "on scene."
- Read the history log on the right side of the screen.
- Perform your assessments and interventions using the buttons in the left panel. When you have determined that it is appropriate to begin transporting your patient to the hospital, click the **Load Patient** button. Continue your assessments and interventions en route to the hospital. When you have finished treating your patient, click the **Unload Patient** button. You will be taken to the summary menu.
- Click the **Log** button on the summary menu, and review your patient care as you answer the following questions.

1. As the paramedics approach Patrick's home, they assess the scene. What are your impressions of the visual assessment of the outside of Patrick's home? What should the paramedics consider based on the assessment of the exterior of Patrick's home?

2. Upon entering Patrick's home, several clues stand out that Patrick may be in trouble on several different levels. List the clues and concerns you would have as you entered Patrick's home.

3. During your assessment of Patrick, you open his shirt to listen for lung sounds and discover a catheter beneath his left clavicle. What might this discovery indicate? What should you do if during assessment you discovered a medication port, such as a portacath?

4. During your assessment of Patrick's arms before taking a blood pressure, you palpate a dialysis shunt. Would you be able to assess a blood pressure on that arm? How would you assess Patrick's blood pressure if dialysis shunts were found in both arms?

5. During your assessment of Patrick's arms before you assess the blood pressure, you palpate a peripherally inserted central catheter (PICC) line. How should the paramedic manage the assessment given this discovery?

6. The paramedic returns after closing the kitchen door and reports that he opened the refrigerator to look for insulin. He reports the refrigerator was unplugged, was warm, and smelled of spoiled food. What does this indicate? Detail how you would question the Patrick about this discovery.

7. While obtaining the SAMPLE history, the paramedic has asked Patrick about the use of medications. He indicates the bottles on the table and states, "That's not all of them." Once most of the medications are collected, the paramedic notes some expired labels, many different prescribing physicians, many different pharmacies, and varying strengths of the same medication. What might this indicate to the paramedic?

8. Patrick has told the paramedic that he may look in the drawer to find additional medications. In the drawer, the paramedic finds an unsigned do not resuscitate form. How should the paramedic approach this discovery with Patrick?

9. During the assessment, the paramedic notes that Patrick is incontinent of urine and stool, and the chair cushion is wet. List some differential diagnoses that may explain why Patrick would have been unable to use the bathroom?

10. If Patrick were found in an assisted-living facility, would the nature of his complaint be an emergency? Suppose the complaint centered around the oxygen bottle needing to be refilled. How should the paramedic address that?

11. Assume one of the medications on the table is Zoloft. What is this medication used for, and would this be expected for Patrick?

12. Complete a patient care report (PCR) for this call. (Use one of the blank PCRs in the back of your study guide or the one your instructor has given you).

- To save your log, click on the disk icon. To print your log, click on the printer icon.
- Click **Menu** to return to the summary menu.
- Click **Exit** to close the program, or **Restart** to continue with another lesson.

Abuse and Assault

👓 **Reading Assignment:** Read Chapter 39, Abuse and Assault, in *Paramedic Practice Today: Above and Beyond*.

Other Relevant Chapters:
- Chapter 4, Legal and Regulatory Issues
- Chapter 8, Pathophysiology
- Chapter 11, Basic Principles of Pharmacology
- Chapter 12, Drug and Chemical Classes
- Chapter 15, Therapeutic Communication
- Chapter 16, History Taking
- Chapter 17, Patient Assessment
- Chapter 19, Documentation
- Chapter 24, Head and Face Trauma
- Chapter 30, Toxicology
- Chapter 45, Soft Tissue Trauma
- Chapter 46, Burn Injury
- Chapter 48, Spinal Trauma
- Chapter 59, Crime Scene Awareness

Case 9: 22-year-old female—assault

Objectives:

On completion of this lesson, the student will be able to perform the following:
- Outline the care for the physical and psychologic needs of a patient who has been subjected to physical, sexual, or emotional abuse.
- Discuss how to integrate principles of crime scene preservation during the assessment and management of a patient who has been subjected to physical, sexual, or emotional abuse.
- Document the call appropriately.

EXERCISE 1

 CD-ROM Activity

 Time: 15 minutes

- Sign into the software by entering your name in the name tag and clicking **Enter.**
- Choose the case by clicking on *Case 9: 22-year-old female—assault.*
- Listen to the dispatch, or read it in the right panel (or both).
- Click **Start** and watch the entire video. Once the video has concluded, you are "on scene."
- Read the history log on the right side of the screen.
- Perform your assessments and interventions using the buttons in the left panel. When you have determined that it is appropriate to begin transporting your patient to the hospital, click the **Load Patient** button. Continue your assessments and interventions en route to the hospital. When you have finished treating your patient, click the **Unload Patient** button. You will be taken to the summary menu.
- Click the **Log** button on the summary menu, and review your patient care as you answer the following questions.

1. Based on the initial information you received from dispatch and your initial assessment, list at least four injuries or illnesses that you may encounter on this call.

2. As you enter the room to assess and manage the patient, what are your priorities?

3. Describe why you believe the patient should or should not have spinal immobilization (spinal motion restriction).

4. Why should you exercise extreme caution if you elect to administer pain medicine to this patient?

5. Describe the detailed assessment you would perform on this patient's jaw.

6. Describe the signs or symptoms that would lead you to suspect that this patient has an inhalation injury?

7. Is a genital examination indicated? Explain your rationale.

8. List the specific injury you suspect and at least one possible complication related to the injuries you observed in the patient on this call.

Sign or Symptom	Specific Injury Suspected	Possible Complications
Burns around the nose or mouth		
Severe pain of the jaw		

9. For each drug that you administered in this case, describe at least two effects it had and the reason for these effects.

Drug	Effect	Explanation
	(1)	(1)
	(2)	(2)
	(1)	(1)
	(2)	(2)

10. Graph the heart rate and oxygen saturation (SaO_2) that you obtained (consult your log). Connect the data points so that each vital sign forms a line (see example). Use blue ink for the heart rate and red ink for SaO_2.

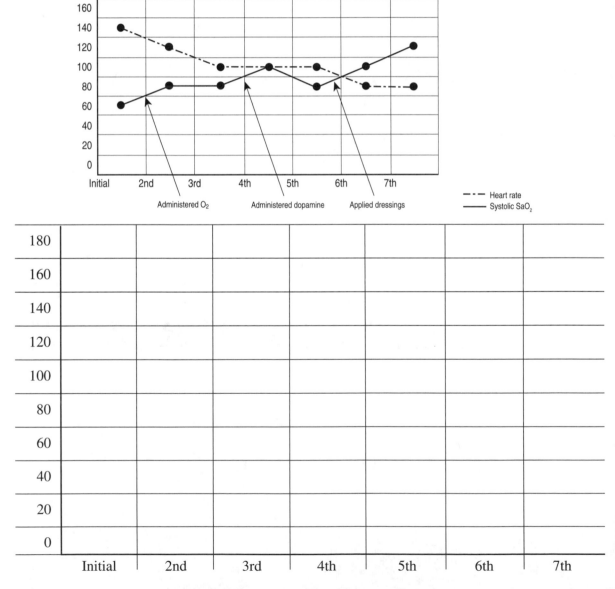

11. Referring to your own graph on the previous page, answer the following questions.

   a. What trends do you observe?

   b. How did your interventions relate to the trends you observe? (You may want to label your graph with interventions performed at various intervals as shown in the example.)

   c. If the trend reversed at any point, how can you explain that variation?

12. Should you ask the police officer to leave so you can protect the patient's rights as granted by the Health Insurance Portability and Accountability Act (HIPAA) of 1996? Explain your answer.

13. Complete a patient care report (PCR) for this call. (Use one of the blank PCRs in the back of your study guide or one your instructor has given you).

→ • To save your log, click on the disk icon. To print your log, click on the printer icon.
   • Click **Menu** to return to the summary menu.
   • Click **Exit** to close the program, or **Restart** to continue with another lesson.

EXERCISE 2

Summary Activity

Time: 15 minutes

14. How do you think you handled this call?

15. Do you think you would change your actions if given the opportunity to complete the call again?

    If you said *yes,* what would you change and how do you think those changes would affect the patient?

→ • Review your call log with your instructor to see how it compares with the recommended care found in the *Implementation Manual.*

16. How did your care compare with what was recommended?

17. After reviewing the call, would you change anything on a subsequent call of this nature?

LESSON 41

Patients with Special Challenges

Reading Assignment: Read Chapter 40, Patients with Special Challenges, in *Paramedic Practice Today: Above and Beyond*.

Case 2: 56-year-old female—fell

Case 3: 7-year-old female—seizure

Case 13: 5-month-old male—unresponsive

Objectives:

On completion of this lesson, the student will be able to perform the following:

- Describe alterations in normal physiologic functions related to selected patients with special challenges.
- Recognize physical attributes consistent with diseases or conditions that create special challenges.
- Outline the modifications in prehospital patient management that may be necessary when dealing with selected patients with special challenges.

EXERCISE 1

 CD-ROM Activity

 Time: 15 minutes

 • Sign into the software by entering your name in the name tag and clicking **Enter.**
• Choose the case by clicking on *Case 2: 56-year-old female—fell.*
• Listen to the dispatch, or read it in the right panel (or both).
• Click **Start** and watch the entire video. Once the video has concluded, you are "on scene."
• Read the history log on the right side of the screen.

1. Assuming that this patient is 5 feet 2 inches tall and weighs 440 pounds, answer the following questions.

 a. Calculate this patient's body mass index (BMI). (Use the information in Box 40-3 on page 196 of your textbook.)

b. In which category does this BMI place her?

i. Healthful:

ii. Moderately overweight:

iii. Severely overweight:

2. List three possible causes for this patient's obesity.

3. What medical conditions should you anticipate in a morbidly obese patient?

4. What modifications may need to be made when performing the physical examination of this patient?

 • Click **Quit Case,** and you will be taken to the summary menu.

EXERCISE 2

 CD-ROM Activity

 Time: 15 minutes

 • Click **Restart** from the summary menu.
- Choose the case by clicking on *Case 3: 7-year-old female—seizure.*
- Listen to the dispatch, or read it in the right panel (or both).
- Click **Start** and watch the entire video. Once the video has concluded, you are "on scene."
- Read the history log on the right side of the screen.

5. This child's parent indicates that the patient has a history of cerebral palsy. What causes cerebral palsy?

6. Distinguish the physical manifestations among the three types of cerebral palsy.

Spastic Paralysis	Athetosis	Ataxia

7. Do all patients with cerebral palsy have severe mental retardation? Explain your answer.

8. What are the considerations for prehospital care of this patient?

 • Click **Quit Case,** and you will be taken to the summary menu.

EXERCISE 3

 CD-ROM Activity

 Time: 15 minutes

 • Click **Restart** from the summary menu.
- Choose the case by clicking on *Case 13: 5-month-old male—unresponsive.*
- Listen to the dispatch, or read it in the right panel (or both).
- Click on **Start** and watch the entire video. Once the video has concluded, you are "on scene."
- Read the history log on the right side of the screen.

9. Your initial observation of this child indicates physical characteristics of Down syndrome. List other physical characteristics that indicate Down syndrome.

10. What physical problems are common in patients with Down syndrome?

11. If you encounter an older patient with Down syndrome, what modifications might you need to make during your initial assessment to accommodate this patient's condition?

➔ • Click **Quit Case,** and you will be taken to the summary menu.
   • Click **Exit** to close the program, or **Restart** to continue with another lesson.

Social Issues

✎ **Reading Assignment:** Read Chapter 41, Social Issues, in *Paramedic Practice Today: Above and Beyond*.

Other Relevant Chapters:

- Chapter 30, Toxicology
- Chapter 32, Psychiatric Disorders and Substance Abuse
- Chapter 39, Abuse and Assault

Case 5: 40-year-old male—vomiting blood

Objectives:

On completion of this lesson, the student will be able to perform the following:

- Discuss the role of the paramedic when encountering patients that are in codependent or violent relationships.
- Describe the role of the paramedic when treating a patient who is homeless.
- Discuss medical and trauma conditions that are common with the homeless population.

EXERCISE 1

 CD-ROM Activity

 Time: 15 minutes

- Sign into the software by entering your name in the name tag and clicking **Enter**.
- Choose the case by clicking on *Case 5: 40-year-old male—vomiting blood*.
- Listen to the dispatch, or read it in the right panel (or both).
- Click **Start** and watch the entire video. Once the video has concluded, you are "on scene."
- Read the history log on the right side of the screen.

1. What clues are presented that indicate this patient may have an addiction?

2. If this patient is homeless, how might his condition be affected? Explain your rationale.

3. What considerations should paramedics have when treating a patient who is poor?

- Click **Quit Case**, and you will be taken to the summary menu.
- Click **Exit** to close the program, or **Restart** to continue with another lesson.

Care for the Patient with a Chronic Illness

/OTZ **Reading Assignment:** Read Chapter 42, Care for the Patient with a Chronic Illness, in *Paramedic Practice Today: Above and Beyond.*

Case 14: 65-year-old male—difficulty breathing `

Objectives:

On completion of this lesson, the student will be able to perform the following:

- Predict oxygen equipment problems that may be encountered by a home care patient.
- Identify resources for the home care patient who has an oxygen equipment problem.

EXERCISE 1

 CD-ROM Activity

Time: 10 minutes

→
- Sign into the software by entering your name in the name tag and clicking **Enter.**
- Choose the case by clicking on *Case 14: 65-year-old male—difficulty breathing.*
- Listen to the dispatch, or read it in the right panel (or both).
- Click **Start** and watch the entire video. Once the video has concluded, you are "on scene."
- Read the history log on the right side of the screen.

1. When you see that the patient is on home oxygen, how does this circumstance contribute to your initial impression of the patient's condition?

2. What type of oxygen supply does this patient have? What are the advantages and disadvantages of this type of supply as compared with an oxygen concentrator?

	Patient's Oxygen	Other
Type		Oxygen concentrator
Advantages		
Disadvantages		

3. If this patient's condition were to improve immediately when you removed his nasal cannula and placed him on your tank and your equipment, what specific equipment problems should you suspect?

4. What will you do if:

   a. This patient calls and says that his oxygen tank will run out in 2 hours:

   b. This patient is on an oxygen concentrator, and the power is out in his home:

   c. This patient is on an oxygen concentrator, and the power is out in your entire district:

   d. This patient comes up to your station and asks you to fill his oxygen tank because his will be empty tomorrow:

e. If you have to transport this patient, you may need to transport the home oxygen cylinder as well to ensure the patient has oxygen on the return trip home. What precautions should you take when transporting a home oxygen supply?

 • Click **Quit Case,** and you will be taken to the summary menu.
• Click **Exit** to close the program, or **Restart** to continue with another lesson.

Trauma Systems and Mechanism of Injury

Reading Assignment: Read Chapter 43, Trauma Systems and Mechanism of Injury, in *Paramedic Practice Today: Above and Beyond.*

Case 7: 8-year-old male—submersion

Case 11: 32-year-old male—gunshot wounds

Objectives:

On completion of this lesson, the student will be able to perform the following:

- Describe how the phases of trauma care relate to a particular case.
- Describe how each component of the trauma system can affect this patient's outcome.
- Relate your knowledge of mechanism of injury to predict possible injury patterns in selected cases.

EXERCISE 1

 CD-ROM Activity

 Time: 15 minutes

- Sign into the software by entering your name in the name tag and clicking **Enter.**
- Choose the case by clicking on *Case 7: 8-year-old male—submersion.*
- Listen to the dispatch, or read it in the right panel (or both).
- Click **Start** and watch the entire video. Once the video has concluded, you are "on scene."
- Read the history log on the right side of the screen.

1. Describe the paramedic's role in each phase of trauma care as it relates to this type of injury.

Phase of Care	Possible Paramedic Actions for This Type of Injury
Before event	
Event	
After event	

2. Explain how each of the following components of a trauma system has the potential to affect this patient's clinical outcome.

Component	Possible Effect on This Patient's Outcome
Injury prevention	
Prehospital care	
Emergency department care	
Interfacility transport	
Definitive care	

Component	Possible Effect on This Patient's Outcome
Trauma critical care	
Rehabilitation	
Data collection and trauma registry	

3. This patient was injured in a vertical fall. The three factors that influence injury in this type of fall are (1) the distance fallen, (2) the body position of the patient on impact, and (3) the type of landing surface. Explain the role of each factor in the injuries that this patient sustained.

Factors That Influence Injury after a Fall	How Do These Factors Influence Injury in This Case?
Distance fallen	

Factors That Influence Injury after a Fall	How Do These Factors Influence Injury in This Case?
Body position	
Type of landing surface	

 • Click **Quit Case,** and you will be taken to the summary menu.

EXERCISE 2

 CD-ROM Activity

 Time: 15 minutes

 • Click **Restart** from the summary menu.
- Choose the case by clicking on *Case 11: 32-year-old male—gunshot wounds.*
- Listen to the dispatch, or read it in the right panel (or both).
- Click **Start** and watch the entire video. Once the video has concluded, you are "on scene."
- Read the history log on the right side of the screen.

4. Describe interventions that may be taken by paramedics to reduce the incidence of death in each period in which trauma deaths occur.

Periods of Trauma Death	Paramedic Interventions to Reduce Incidence of Deaths
Immediate	

Periods of Trauma Death	Paramedic Interventions to Reduce Incidence of Deaths
Early	
Late	

5. Kinetic energy is equal to one-half the mass multiplied by the velocity squared:

$$KE = (m/2) \times V^2$$

Explain the factors in a shooting that influence tissue damage as they relate to this formula.

→ • Click **Quit Case,** and you will be taken to the summary menu.
   • Click **Exit** to close the program, or **Restart** to continue with another lesson.

Multisystem Trauma

Reading Assignment: Read Chapter 44, Bleeding; Chapter 45, Soft Tissue Trauma, Chapter 47, Head and Face Trauma; Chapter 48, Spinal Trauma; Chapter 49, Thoracic Trauma; Chapter 50, Abdominal Trauma; and Chapter 51, Musculoskeletal Trauma, in *Paramedic Practice Today: Above and Beyond.*

Other Relevant Chapters:
- Chapter 1, EMS Safety and Well-Being of the Paramedic
- Chapter 4, Legal and Regulatory Issues
- Chapter 7, Body Systems: Anatomy and Physiology
- Chapter 8, Pathophysiology
- Chapter 13, Medication Administration
- Chapter 14, Airway Management
- Chapter 16, History Taking
- Chapter 17, Patient Assessment
- Chapter 19, Documentation
- Chapter 43, Trauma Systems and Mechanism of Injury
- Chapter 59, Crime Scene Awareness

Case 11: 32-year-old male—gunshot wounds

Objectives:
On completion of this lesson, the student will be able to perform the following:
- Demonstrate appropriate actions to take when responding to a patient injured by gunshots.
- Predict the injuries from penetrating trauma based on knowledge of anatomy and physiology.
- Manage life threats, including airway, breathing, and circulatory problems, for the patient with penetrating trauma.
- Document the call appropriately.

EXERCISE 1

   CD-ROM Activity

Time: 25 minutes

- Sign into the software by entering your name in the name tag and clicking **Enter.**
- Choose the case by clicking on *Case 11: 32-year-old male—gunshot wounds.*
- Listen to the dispatch, or read it in the right panel (or both).
- Click **Start** and watch the entire video. Once the video has concluded, you are "on scene."

1. How do you know that the scene is safe and you may approach the patient?

- Read the history log on the right side of the screen.
- Perform your assessments and interventions using the buttons in the left panel. When you have determined that it is appropriate to begin transporting your patient to the hospital, click the **Load Patient** button. Continue your assessments and interventions en route to the hospital. When you have finished treating your patient, click the **Unload Patient** button. You will be taken to the summary menu.
- Click the **Log** button on the summary menu, and review your patient care as you answer the following questions.

2. What immediate life threats did you identify in this patient?

3. What type of dressing would you apply to each wound? Discuss your rationale for the application of each.

Wound	Dressing	Rationale
Neck		
Chest		
Abdomen		

4. List three causes of shock that you identified in this patient. What signs, symptoms, or physical findings led you to the clinical impression in each case? How did each type of shock affect preload?

Type of Shock	Signs, Symptoms, and Findings That Suggest This Type of Shock	Effect on Preload

5. Explain the rationale for the airway, ventilation, and oxygenation choices you made for this patient.

6. Based on the location of the gunshot wounds and the patient's signs and symptoms, predict which organs or significant body structures each bullet injured.

   a. Neck:

   b. Chest:

   c. Abdomen:

7. List at least three measures you should take to preserve evidence on this call.

8. Complete a patient care report (PCR) for this call. (Use one of the blank PCRs in the back of your study guide or the one your instructor has given you.)

- To save your log, click on the disk icon. To print your log, click on the printer icon.
- Click **Quit Case** and you will be taken to the summary menu.
- Click **Exit** to close the program, or **Restart** to continue with another lesson.

EXERCISE 2

Summary Activity

Time: 15 minutes

9. How did you feel about how you handled this call?

10. Do you think you would change your actions if given the opportunity to complete the call again?

If you said *yes,* what would you change and how do you think those changes would affect the patient?

→ • Review your log with your instructor to see how it compares with the recommended care found in the *Implementation Manual*.

11. How did your care compare with what was recommended?

12. After reviewing the call, would you change anything on a subsequent call of this kind? Explain your answer.

Burn Injury

Reading Assignment: Read Chapter 46, Burn Injury, in *Paramedic Practice Today: Above and Beyond*.

Case 9: 22-year-old female—assault

Objectives:

On completion of this lesson, the student will be able to perform the following:

- Apply knowledge of factors that influence the severity of a burn injury to predict the mechanism of injury in this case.
- Classify burn injuries according to depth, extent, and severity.
- Predict signs and symptoms a patient with a burn injury may exhibit, based on the pathophysiologic understanding of a burn injury.
- Calculate fluid volume requirements for selected burn injury cases.

EXERCISE 1

  CD-ROM Activity

 Time: 15 minutes

→ • Sign into the software by entering your name in the name tag and clicking **Enter.**
  • Choose the case by clicking on *Case 9: 22-year-old female—assault.*
  • Listen to the dispatch, or read it in the right panel (or both).
  • Click **Start** and watch the entire video. Once the video has concluded, you are "on scene."
  • Read the history log on the right side of the screen.

1. Predict whether the severity of burn injury would have been more or less had this patient been 85 years of age. Explain your answer.

2. Describe the pathophysiologic mechanisms that create the blisters found in partial thickness burns.

3. Does the patient have injuries that meet the criteria for referral to a burn center? Explain your answer.

4. Use the Consensus Burn Formula on page 367 in Chapter 46 of your textbook to calculate the fluid replacement requirements in the first hour after a burn injury for each of the following patient examples. Calculate the drops per minute in each example, based on the intravenous (IV) tubing drop factor.

Patient Weight	Percent Body Surface Area Burned			Total Volume to Infuse in First Hour after Burn	IV Tubing Drop Factor (gtt/mL)	Drops per Minute to Regulate IV Fluids
	Superficial	Partial Thickness	Full Thickness			
a. 60 lb	0%	0%	40%		20	
b. 90 lb	0%	10%	40%		15	
c. 150 lb	10%	40%	30%		10	
d. 240 lb	30%	20%	30%		10	

5. Explain the pathophysiologic significance of a circumferential full-thickness burn in each of the following body regions.

   a. Neck:

   b. Upper arm:

   c. Chest:

- Click **Quit Case,** and you will be taken to the summary menu.
- Click **Exit** to close the program, or **Restart** to continue with another lesson.

LESSON 47

Environmental Conditions

👓 **Reading Assignment:** Read Chapter 52, Environmental Conditions, in *Paramedic Practice Today: Above and Beyond*.

Other Relevant Chapters:
- Chapter 13, Medication Administration
- Chapter 16, History Taking
- Chapter 17, Patient Assessment
- Chapter 19, Documentation
- Chapter 22, Cardiovascular Disorders
- Chapter 24, Endocrine Emergencies and Nutritional Disorders
- Chapter 55, Assessment-Based Management
- Chapter 61, Emergency Vehicle Operations

Case 12: 57-year-old male—man down

Objectives:

On completion of this lesson, the student will be able to perform the following:
- Interpret information from the patient history and physical examination to form the appropriate clinical impression.
- Perform interventions sequentially, and revise the treatment plan based on feedback from an appropriate reassessment.

EXERCISE 1

 CD-ROM Activity

 Time: 15 minutes

- Sign into the software by entering your name in the name tag and clicking **Enter.**
- Choose the case by clicking on *Case 12: 57-year-old male—man down.*
- Listen to the dispatch, or read it in the right panel (or both).
- Click **Start** and watch the entire video. Once the video has concluded, you are "on scene."
- Read the history log on the right side of the screen.
- Perform your assessments and interventions using the buttons in the left panel. When you have determined that it is appropriate to begin transporting your patient to the hospital, click the **Load Patient** button. Continue your assessments and interventions en route to the hospital. When you have finished treating your patient, click the **Unload Patient** button. You will be taken to the summary menu.
- Click the **Log** button on the summary menu, and review your patient care as you answer the following questions.

1. What ECG rhythm did you initially observe?

2. Explain the pathophysiologic cause of that rhythm.

3. Explain why you selected the oxygen device and flow rate that you did.

4. What noninvasive interventions should you perform before transporting? Explain the rationale for performing these interventions.

5. Identify preexisting illnesses or conditions that placed this patient at high risk for his present illness? Why did these conditions predispose him to this illness?

Preexisting Condition	Rationale

6. Explain the following pathophysiologic signs or symptoms and how they work to compensate for the patient's illness.

Sign or Symptom	Mechanism of Compensation
Diaphoresis	
Respiratory rate of 32 breaths/min	

7. If you fail to intervene in a timely manner for this patient, predict the progression of his illness.

8. If the patient begins to shiver:

   a. Explain the physiologic consequences that this sign might produce.

   b. Describe treatment measures you would use.

9. What environmental factors contribute to this type of illness?

10. Graph the systolic blood pressure (BP) and heart rate that you obtained in this call (consult your log). Then connect the data points so that each vital sign forms a line (see example). You can use blue ink for the systolic BP and red ink for the heart rate.

11. Referring to your own graph, answer the following questions:

    a. What trends do you observe?

    b. How did your interventions relate to the trends you observed? (You may want to label your graph with interventions performed at various intervals as shown in the example.)

    c. If the trend reversed at any point, how can you explain that variation?

12. Complete a patient care report (PCR) for this call. (Use one of the blank PCRs in the back of your study guide or one your instructor has given you.)

- To save your log, click on the disk icon. To print your log, click on the printer icon.
- Click **Menu** to return to the summary menu.
- Click **Exit** to close the program, or **Restart** to continue with another lesson.

EXERCISE 2

Summary Activity

Time: 15 minutes

13. How did you feel about how you handled this call?

14. Do you think you would change your actions if given the opportunity to complete the call again?

    If you said *yes,* what would you change and how do you think those changes would affect the patient?

 • Review your log with your instructor to see how it compares with the recommended care found in the *Implementation Manual.*

15. How did your care compare with what was recommended?

16. After reviewing the call, would you change anything on a subsequent call of this nature?

Assessment-Based Management

Reading Assignment: Read Chapter 55, Assessment-Based Management, in *Paramedic Practice Today: Above and Beyond*.

Case 1: 20-year-old male—difficulty breathing

Case 2: 56-year-old female—fell

Case 6: 16-year-old female—unknown medical

Case 7: 8-year-old male—submersion

Case 8: 38-year-old male—suicide attempt

Case 12: 57-year-old male—man down

Objectives:

On completion of this lesson, the student will be able to perform the following:

- Use *pattern recognition* to assess and treat each of the cases in this chapter.
- Form a field impression of the patient presented in each case, then develop and carry out a plan of action.

EXERCISE 1

 CD-ROM Activity

 Time: 15 minutes

→
- Sign into the software by entering your name in the name tag and clicking **Enter.**
- Choose the case by clicking on *Case 1: 20-year-old male—difficulty breathing.*
- Listen to the dispatch, or read it in the right panel (or both).
- Click **Start** and watch the entire video. Once the video has concluded, you are "on scene."
- Read the history log on the right side of the screen.
- Perform your initial assessment using the **Assessment** buttons in the left panel.

1. Has adequate information been provided by the resident advisor and firefighters to form a working field impression?

2. What is your field impression of James's illness? Defend your answer.

3. Is it possible that James may be suffering from more than one illness? What illness or illnesses do you suspect? Explain.

4. Based on your assessment and field impression, detail your action plan for James.

→
- Click **Quit Case,** and you will be taken to the summary menu.

EXERCISE 2

 CD-ROM Activity

 Time: 15 minutes

- Click **Restart** from the summary menu.
- Choose the case by clicking on *Case 2: 56-year-old female—fell.*
- Listen to the dispatch, or read it in the right panel (or both).
- Click **Start** and watch the entire video. Once the video has concluded, you are "on scene."
- Read the history log on the right side of the screen.
- Perform your initial assessment using the **Assessment** buttons in the left panel.

5. Does the woman's husband provide enough information to formulate a working field assessment?

6. What attitude might the paramedic have to overcome to deal effectively with this patient?

7. What is your field impression of this patient?

8. Based on your assessment and field impression, detail your action plan for this patient.

- Click **Quit Case,** and you will be taken to the summary menu.

EXERCISE 3

 CD-ROM Activity

 Time: 10 minutes

• Click **Restart** from the summary menu.
• Choose the case by clicking on *Case 6: 16-year-old female—unknown medical.*
• Listen to the dispatch, or read it in the right panel (or both).
• Click **Start** and watch the entire video. Once the video has concluded, you are "on scene."
• Read the history log on the right side of the screen.

9. What is your initial impression of this patient?

10. What are your safety concerns about this patient?

11. What is your field impression of this patient?

• Click **Quit Case,** and you will be taken to the summary menu.

EXERCISE 4

 CD-ROM Activity

 Time: 15 minutes

- Click **Restart** from the summary menu.
- Choose the case by clicking on *Case 7: 8-year-old male—submersion.*
- Listen to the dispatch, or read it in the right panel (or both).
- Click **Start** and watch the entire video. Once the video has concluded, you are "on scene."
- Read the history log on the right side of the screen.
- Perform your initial assessment using the **Assessment** buttons in the left panel.

12. Would the initial approach to this patient change if he were still in the pool? Explain.

13. What is your field impression of this patient?

14. Based on your field impression and initial assessment of this patient, detail your plan of action in order of importance.

15. Where should this patient be transported? Explain.

- Click **Quit Case,** and you will be taken to the summary menu.

EXERCISE 5

 CD-ROM Activity

 Time: 10 minutes

- Click **Restart** from the summary menu.
- Choose the case by clicking on *Case 8: 38-year-old male—suicide attempt*.
- Listen to the dispatch, or read it in the right panel (or both).
- Click **Start** and watch the entire video. Once the video has concluded, you are "on scene."
- Read the history log on the right side of the screen.
- Perform your initial assessment using the **Assessment** buttons in the left panel.

16. What is your field impression of Robbie?

17. What are some differential diagnoses for Robbie's behavior?

18. How would your approach to Robbie change if the police officer had "tased" him?

19. Based on your field impression and assessment, detail a plan of action for Robbie.

→ • Click **Quit Case,** and you will be taken to the summary menu.

EXERCISE 6

 CD-ROM Activity

 Time: 10 minutes

- Click **Restart** from the summary menu.
- Choose the case by clicking on *Case 12: 57-year-old male—man down.*
- Listen to the dispatch, or read it in the right panel (or both).
- Click **Start** and watch the entire video. Once the video has concluded, you are "on scene."
- Read the history log on the right side of the screen.
- Perform your initial assessment using the **Assessment** buttons in the left panel.

20. What is your initial impression of Ted?

21. What extenuating circumstances need to be considered during your assessment?

22. Does Ted have risk factors for cardiac disease? If so, what are they?

23. What are some differential diagnoses for Ted's signs and symptoms?

- Click **Quit Case,** and you will be taken to the summary menu.
- Click **Exit** to close the program, or **Restart** to continue with another lesson.

Clinical Decision Making

Reading Assignment: Read Chapter 56, Clinical Decision Making, in *Paramedic Practice Today: Above and Beyond.*

Case 15: 42-year-old male—difficulty breathing

Case 2: 56-year-old female—fell

Objectives:

On completion of this lesson, the student will be able to perform the following:

- Apply clinical decision making tools to selected virtual patient encounters (VPE).

- Outline the elements of clinical decision making in emergency medical services (EMS) scenarios.

EXERCISE 1

 CD-ROM Activity

 Time: 15 minutes

- Sign into the software by entering your name in the name tag and clicking **Enter.**
- Choose the case by clicking on *Case 15: 42-year-old male—difficulty breathing.*
- Listen to the dispatch, or read it in the right panel (or both).
- Click **Start** and watch the entire video. Once the video has concluded, you are "on scene."
- Read the history log on the right side of the screen.
- Perform your assessments and interventions using the buttons in the left panel. When you have determined that it is appropriate to begin transporting your patient to the hospital, click the **Load Patient** button. Continue your assessments and interventions en route to the hospital. When you have finished treating your patient, click the **Unload Patient** button. You will be taken to the summary menu.
- Click the **Log** button on the summary menu, and review your patient care as you answer the following questions.

1. Below are the steps in the clinical decision-making process. What did you assess or do in each area (if anything) on this call, and what were your findings and actions?

Elements of Decision Making	Steps in Process	Findings and Actions
Read the scene		
Read the patient		
React		

Elements of Decision Making	Steps in Process	Findings and Actions
Reevaluate		
Revise the treatment plan		
Review performance at the run critique		

2. Why is it difficult to make a clear treatment decision concerning this patient?

3. What information helped your formation of the concept in this case?

4. Was there an algorithm or distinct treatment path that resolved this patient's crisis in the field? Explain your answer.

• To save your log, click on the disk icon. To print your log, click on the printer icon.
• Click **Menu** to return to the summary menu.

EXERCISE 2

 CD-ROM Activity

 Time: 15 minutes

 • Click **Restart** from the summary menu.
• Choose the case by clicking on *Case 2: 56-year-old female—fell.*
• Listen to the dispatch, or read it in the right panel (or both).
• Click **Start** and watch the entire video. Once the video has concluded, you are "on scene."
• Read the history log on the right side of the screen.

5. What information on this call became barriers to the formation of your initial concept?

6. What features in the practice environment on this case increased the challenges of caring for this patient?

7. When you viewed the initial video and had the information it presented, did you have sufficient data to place the patient's care into a standard treatment algorithm? Explain your answer.

 • Click **Quit Case,** and you will be taken to the summary menu.
• Click **Exit** to close the program, or **Restart** to continue with another lesson.

Crime Scene Awareness

/Oᴆᴅ **Reading Assignment:** Read Chapter 59, Crime Scene Awareness, in *Paramedic Practice Today: Above and Beyond.*

Case 11: 32-year-old male—gunshot wounds

Case 14: 65-year-old male—difficulty breathing

Case 3: 7-year-old female—seizing

Objectives:

On completion of this lesson, the student will be able to perform the following:

- Identify paramedic practices to promote safety on a crime scene.
- Distinguish between cover and concealment.

EXERCISE 1

 CD-ROM Activity

 Time: 15 minutes

- Sign into the software by entering your name in the name tag and clicking **Enter.**
- Choose the case by clicking on *Case 11: 32-year-old male—gunshot wounds.*
- Listen to the dispatch, or read it in the right panel (or both).
- Click **Start** and watch the entire video. Once the video has concluded, you are "on scene."

1. Describe where you should stage the ambulance on this call if a concern exists regarding scene safety.

2. Look around the environment.

    a. To where would you run to seek cover?

    b. Where would you go for concealment?

→ • Click **Quit Case,** and go to the summary menu.

EXERCISE 2

  CD-ROM Activity

 Time: 15 minutes

- Click **Restart** from the summary menu.
- Choose the case by clicking on *Case 14: 65-year-old male—difficulty breathing.*
- Listen to the dispatch, or read it in the right panel (or both).
- Click **Start** and watch the entire video. Once the video has concluded, you are "on scene."

3. Would the approach to the door by the emergency medical services (EMS) crew be acceptable if this scene were considered unsafe? Explain your answer.

4. If you needed to retreat suddenly outside the house because a dangerous person with a gun was pursuing you, where would you seek:

   a. Concealment:

   b. Cover:

- Click **Quit Case,** and you will be taken to the summary menu.

EXERCISE 3

 CD-ROM Activity

 Time: 10 minutes

- Click **Restart** from the summary menu.
- Chose the case by clicking on *Case 3: 7-year-old female—seizing*.
- Listen to the dispatch, or read it in the right panel (or both).
- Click **Start** and watch the entire video. Once the video has concluded, you are "on scene."

5. Because the room the patient is occupying does not provide an escape route for paramedics in the event that the father becomes violent, what should paramedics do?

- Click **Quit Case**, and you will be taken to the summary menu.
- Click **Exit** to close the program, or **Restart** to continue with another lesson.

LESSON 51

Dispatch Activities

Reading Assignment: Read Chapter 60, Dispatch Activities, in *Paramedic Practice Today: Above and Beyond*.

Case 1: 20-year-old male—difficulty breathing

Case 7: 8-year-old male—submersion

Case 13: 5-month-old male—unresponsive

Case 2: 56-year-old female—fell

Case 10: 25-year-old female—abdominal pain

Objectives:

On completion of this lesson, the student will be able to perform the following:

• Explain the role of dispatch in the EMS response.

• Describe how chief complaint information determines the resources deployed in the response.

• Explain how systematic questioning can improve the quality of information obtained by the dispatcher.

EXERCISE 1

  CD-ROM Activity

 Time: 20 minutes

 • Sign into the software by entering your name in the name tag and clicking **Enter**.

1. *Response prioritization and resource alignment plan:* Listen to the dispatch information for Case 1, Case 7, and Case 13. Why did the dispatcher send an engine company on these calls? What information might they have received that indicated the need for an engine company?

 • Choose the case by clicking on *Case 1: 20-year-old-male—difficulty breathing*.
• Listen to the dispatch, or read it in the right panel (or both)

   a. Case 1: 20-year-old-male—difficulty breathing:

 • Click **Quit Case**, and you will be returned to the summary screen.
• Click **Restart** from the summary menu.
• Choose the case by clicking on *Case 7: 8 year-old-male—submersion*.
• Listen to the dispatch, or read it in the right panel (or both)

   b. Case 7: 8-year-old-male—submersion:

- Click **Quit Case**, and you will be returned to the summary screen.
- Click **Restart** from the summary menu.
- Choose the case by clicking on *Case 13: 5-month-old-male—unresponsive*.
- Listen to the dispatch, or read it in the right panel (or both)

    c. Case 13: 5 month-old-male—unresponsive:

- Click **Quit Case**, and you will be returned to the summary screen.
- Click **Restart** from the summary menu.
- Choose the case by clicking on *Case 2: 56-year-old female—fell*.
- Listen to the dispatch, or read it in the right panel (or both)

2. Listen to the dispatch information for Case 2 and compare the information the dispatcher provides with the information found by the paramedics on the scene. Why did the call come in as a fall and not as difficulty breathing and chest pain?

- Click **Quit Case**, and you will be returned to the summary screen.

EXERCISE 2

  CD-ROM Activity

Time: 10 minutes

- Click **Restart** from the summary menu.
- Choose the case by clicking on *Case 10: 25 year-old-female—abdominal pain*.
- Listen to the dispatch, or read it in the right panel (or both)

3. Listen to the call information provided by the dispatcher. Why are the directions more detailed on this call than on any of the other calls?

- Click **Quit Case**, and you will be returned to the summary screen.
- Click **Exit** to close the program, or **Restart** to continue with another lesson.

52 _____

Emergency Vehicle Operations

_____

👓 **Reading Assignment:** Read Chapter 57, Ground and Air Transport of Critical Patients; and Chapter 61, Emergency Vehicle Operations in *Paramedic Practice Today: Above and Beyond.*

Case 5: 40-year-old male—vomiting blood

Objectives:

On completion of this lesson, the student will be able to perform the following:

- Relate the need for specialty resources to this case.
- Describe appropriate helicopter safety procedures as they relate to this case.

EXERCISE 1

 CD-ROM Activity

 Time: 10 minutes

- Sign into the software by entering your name in the name tag and clicking **Enter.**
- Choose the case by clicking on *Case 5: 40-year-old male—vomiting blood.*
- Listen to the dispatch, or read it in the right panel (or both).
- Click **Start** and watch the entire video. Once the video has concluded, you are "on scene."
- Read the history log on the right side of the screen.

1. Does this call meet the general requirements for air medical transport? Explain your answer.

2. Are there specific requirements for air medical transport in your local region that you would take into consideration on this call?

3. Can you identify a suitable landing zone, based on what you saw in the video?

4. What additional resources might be needed to set up the landing zone?

5. When you examine the site you selected, and if time is available, what measures should be taken to make the landing zone safer?

6. If the air ambulance is not available, should you transport the patient with or without lights and sirens? Explain your answer.

7. Describe how you will proceed through intersections.

8. What are the laws in your state as they apply to ambulance operations in emergency mode?

→ • Click **Quit Case,** and you will be taken to the summary menu.
  • Click **Exit** to close the program, or **Restart** to continue with another lesson.

Vehicle Rescue and Rescue Awareness and Operations

Reading Assignment: Read Chapter 63, Vehicle Rescue and Rescue Awareness and Operations, in *Paramedic Practice Today: Above and Beyond*.

Case 8: 38-year-old male—suicide attempt

Objectives:

On completion of this lesson, the student will be able to perform the following:

- Identify specialized resources needed for a rescue on a hazardous terrain.
- Discuss techniques to conduct a rescue on a hazardous terrain.

EXERCISE 1

 CD-ROM Activity

 Time: 10 minutes

- Sign into the software by entering your name in the name tag and clicking **Enter.**
- Choose the case by clicking on *Case 8: 38-year-old male—suicide attempt*.
- Listen to the dispatch, or read it in the right panel (or both).
- Click **Start** and watch the entire video. Once the video has concluded, you are "on scene."
- Read the history log on the right side of the screen.

1. Assume that this patient jumped and was injured in his fall off of the cliff. What additional resources would you need to call?

2. What type of rescue would be involved to get him up the cliff if no access is provided from the bottom?

3. What specific resource would be called in your local area?

4. What type of specialized equipment might be needed to get the patient up from the bottom of the cliff?

5. Should you immediately go to care for the patient at the bottom of the cliff?

6. If you are able to access the patient to evaluate and treat him at the bottom of the cliff, what special considerations might you need to take into account?

 • Click **Quit Case** and you will be taken to the summary menu.
• Click **Exit** to close the program, or **Restart** to continue with another lesson.

Patient Care Report Blanks

CASE 1

CHIEF COMPLAINT	
CURRENT MEDICATIONS	☐ NONE KNOWN
ALLERGIES (MEDICATIONS)	☐ NONE KNOWN
MEDICAL HISTORY	☐ MI ☐ CHF ☐ COPD ☐ ↑ BP ☐ DIABETES ☐ CANCER ☐ NONE KNOWN ☐ OTHER
NARRATIVE	

TIME	P	R	B/P	RHYTHM	TREATMENT	RESPONSE/COMMENTS

CASE 2

CHIEF COMPLAINT	
CURRENT MEDICATIONS	☐ NONE KNOWN
ALLERGIES (MEDICATIONS)	☐ NONE KNOWN
MEDICAL HISTORY	☐ MI ☐ CHF ☐ COPD ☐ ↑ BP ☐ DIABETES ☐ CANCER ☐ NONE KNOWN ☐ OTHER
NARRATIVE	

TIME	P	R	B/P	RHYTHM	TREATMENT	RESPONSE/COMMENTS

CASE 3

CHIEF COMPLAINT	
CURRENT MEDICATIONS	☐ NONE KNOWN
ALLERGIES (MEDICATIONS)	☐ NONE KNOWN
MEDICAL HISTORY	☐ MI ☐ CHF ☐ COPD ☐ ↑ BP ☐ DIABETES ☐ CANCER ☐ NONE KNOWN ☐ OTHER
NARRATIVE	

TIME	P	R	B/P	RHYTHM	TREATMENT	RESPONSE/COMMENTS

CASE 4

CHIEF COMPLAINT	
CURRENT MEDICATIONS	☐ NONE KNOWN
ALLERGIES (MEDICATIONS)	☐ NONE KNOWN
MEDICAL HISTORY	☐ MI ☐ CHF ☐ COPD ☐ ↑ BP ☐ DIABETES ☐ CANCER ☐ NONE KNOWN ☐ OTHER
NARRATIVE	

TIME	P	R	B/P	RHYTHM	TREATMENT	RESPONSE/COMMENTS

CASE 5

CHIEF COMPLAINT	
CURRENT MEDICATIONS	☐ NONE KNOWN
ALLERGIES (MEDICATIONS)	☐ NONE KNOWN
MEDICAL HISTORY	☐ MI ☐ CHF ☐ COPD ☐ ↑ BP ☐ DIABETES ☐ CANCER ☐ NONE KNOWN ☐ OTHER
NARRATIVE	

TIME	P	R	B/P	RHYTHM	TREATMENT	RESPONSE/COMMENTS

CASE 6

CHIEF COMPLAINT	
CURRENT MEDICATIONS	☐ NONE KNOWN
ALLERGIES (MEDICATIONS)	☐ NONE KNOWN
MEDICAL HISTORY	☐ MI ☐ CHF ☐ COPD ☐ ↑ BP ☐ DIABETES ☐ CANCER ☐ NONE KNOWN ☐ OTHER
NARRATIVE	

TIME	P	R	B/P	RHYTHM	TREATMENT	RESPONSE/COMMENTS

CASE 7

CHIEF COMPLAINT	
CURRENT MEDICATIONS	☐ NONE KNOWN
ALLERGIES (MEDICATIONS)	☐ NONE KNOWN
MEDICAL HISTORY	☐ MI ☐ CHF ☐ COPD ☐ ↑ BP ☐ DIABETES ☐ CANCER ☐ NONE KNOWN ☐ OTHER
NARRATIVE	

TIME	P	R	B/P	RHYTHM	TREATMENT	RESPONSE/COMMENTS

CASE 8

CHIEF COMPLAINT	
CURRENT MEDICATIONS	☐ NONE KNOWN
ALLERGIES (MEDICATIONS)	☐ NONE KNOWN
MEDICAL HISTORY	☐ MI ☐ CHF ☐ COPD ☐ ↑ BP ☐ DIABETES ☐ CANCER ☐ NONE KNOWN ☐ OTHER
NARRATIVE	

TIME	P	R	B/P	RHYTHM	TREATMENT	RESPONSE/COMMENTS

CASE 9

CHIEF COMPLAINT	
CURRENT MEDICATIONS	☐ NONE KNOWN
ALLERGIES (MEDICATIONS)	☐ NONE KNOWN
MEDICAL HISTORY	☐ MI ☐ CHF ☐ COPD ☐ ↑ BP ☐ DIABETES ☐ CANCER ☐ NONE KNOWN ☐ OTHER
NARRATIVE	

TIME	P	R	B/P	RHYTHM	TREATMENT	RESPONSE/COMMENTS

CASE 10

CHIEF COMPLAINT	
CURRENT MEDICATIONS	☐ NONE KNOWN
ALLERGIES (MEDICATIONS)	☐ NONE KNOWN
MEDICAL HISTORY	☐ MI ☐ CHF ☐ COPD ☐ ↑ BP ☐ DIABETES ☐ CANCER ☐ NONE KNOWN ☐ OTHER
NARRATIVE	

TIME	P	R	B/P	RHYTHM	TREATMENT	RESPONSE/COMMENTS

CASE 11

CHIEF COMPLAINT	
CURRENT MEDICATIONS	☐ NONE KNOWN
ALLERGIES (MEDICATIONS)	☐ NONE KNOWN
MEDICAL HISTORY	☐ MI ☐ CHF ☐ COPD ☐ ↑ BP ☐ DIABETES ☐ CANCER ☐ NONE KNOWN ☐ OTHER
NARRATIVE	

TIME	P	R	B/P	RHYTHM	TREATMENT	RESPONSE/COMMENTS

CASE 12

CHIEF COMPLAINT	
CURRENT MEDICATIONS	☐ NONE KNOWN
ALLERGIES (MEDICATIONS)	☐ NONE KNOWN
MEDICAL HISTORY	☐ MI ☐ CHF ☐ COPD ☐ ↑ BP ☐ DIABETES ☐ CANCER ☐ NONE KNOWN ☐ OTHER
NARRATIVE	

TIME	P	R	B/P	RHYTHM	TREATMENT	RESPONSE/COMMENTS

CASE 13

CHIEF COMPLAINT	
CURRENT MEDICATIONS	☐ NONE KNOWN
ALLERGIES (MEDICATIONS)	☐ NONE KNOWN
MEDICAL HISTORY	☐ MI ☐ CHF ☐ COPD ☐ ↑ BP ☐ DIABETES ☐ CANCER ☐ NONE KNOWN ☐ OTHER
NARRATIVE	

TIME	P	R	B/P	RHYTHM	TREATMENT	RESPONSE/COMMENTS

CASE 14

CHIEF COMPLAINT	
CURRENT MEDICATIONS	☐ NONE KNOWN
ALLERGIES (MEDICATIONS)	☐ NONE KNOWN
MEDICAL HISTORY	☐ MI ☐ CHF ☐ COPD ☐ ↑ BP ☐ DIABETES ☐ CANCER ☐ NONE KNOWN ☐ OTHER
NARRATIVE	

TIME	P	R	B/P	RHYTHM	TREATMENT	RESPONSE/COMMENTS

CASE 15

CHIEF COMPLAINT	
CURRENT MEDICATIONS	☐ NONE KNOWN
ALLERGIES (MEDICATIONS)	☐ NONE KNOWN
MEDICAL HISTORY	☐ MI ☐ CHF ☐ COPD ☐ ↑ BP ☐ DIABETES ☐ CANCER ☐ NONE KNOWN ☐ OTHER
NARRATIVE	

TIME	P	R	B/P	RHYTHM	TREATMENT	RESPONSE/COMMENTS

Illustration Credits

Lesson 23

Figure with Question 8 adapted from Fig. 9-7 in Phalen T, Aehlert B: *The 12-Lead ECG in Acute Coronary Syndromes,* 2nd ed, 2006, St. Louis, Mosby.

Figure with Question 10 adapted from Box 19-8 in Sanders MJ: *Mosby's Paramedic Textbook,* revised 3rd ed, 2007, St. Louis, Mosby.

Lesson 24

Figure with Question 5 adapted from Fig. 9-53 in Phalen T, Aehlert B: *The 12-Lead ECG in Acute Coronary Syndromes,* 2nd ed, 2006, St. Louis, Mosby.

Lesson 29

Figure with Question 4 adapted from Fig. 14-6 in Huszar RJ: *Basic Dysrhythmias: Interpretation & Management,* revised 3rd edition, 2007, St. Louis, MosbyJems.